When I started to get into the world of nutritional medicine and the work of Dr. Weston Price, DDS, some 20 years ago, I had no idea where it would lead. Now, as the work has grown, particularly with the publication of *Nourishing Traditions* by Sally Fallon, the horizons seem to be rapidly expanding. This work by Kathy Pirtle, Sally Fallon and Dr. Turner expands greatly the use of traditional diets in the treatment of people that I had previously not considered. I, of course, knew the benefits of this approach for many people and types of maladies, but I had never considered the special situation of musicians, dancers and athletes and their musculo-skeletal issues. This well-written and interesting book expands the uses of traditional diets and is a welcome addition to the growing literature on the uses of this approach.

Thomas Cowan, MD
Author of *The Fourfold Path to Healing*

As a close colleague and friend for many years, I have witnessed Kathy Pirtle's transformation—an incredible journey from years of living and performing with pain to vibrant health and career success. The story of a brilliant clarinetist provides a wonderful life lesson of nutrition, full of practical guidance paired with the most advanced nutritional research based on accurate historical data about the diets of healthy populations worldwide. This book is a step beyond anything you have ever read. You will learn the precise principles of optimal nutrition in an easy-to-follow system to help you achieve *your* perfect balance for top performance. A very fun, easy and most interesting read! A *must* for performers and anyone who desires to achieve a higher level of health.

Florentina Ramniceanu
Concertmaster, Chicago Opera Theatre
Violinist, Orion Ensemble

. . . if you're dealing with chronic injury or pain, this is a *"must-read"* for you!

Charlene Zimmerman
Principal Clarinet, Lyric Opera of Chicago
and Grant Park Symphony

This book is a "must-read," from a mother's point of view to that of a professor. Through research from personal health problems, Kathy Pirtle has written a very important and revealing book. The chapter on milk and grass-fed animals just made me smile, since I grew up on raw milk. From a healthy child with no digestive problems to an adult with colitis, I certainly will be researching changes in my diet. From the perspective of a professor, this book also offers new insight into treatment approaches of embouchure strength and stability problems in brass and woodwind players.

Gail Williams
Horn Soloist
Professor of Music, Northwestern University
Former Associate Principal Horn,
Chicago Symphony Orchestra

Who would ever believe that musicians, especially classical musicians, would confront real and at times severe occupational hazards from playing their instruments? But, alas, it is often so. I have personally experienced these myself and have seen careers often end prematurely because performers' bodies just could no longer cope with the pain or discomfort that can follow a serious and relentless pursuit of musical perfection. This book will educate us all and give guidelines that may help others avoid the pitfalls that Ms. Pritle and no doubt others have fallen into. Even if one does not choose to apply this wisdom to one's own particular situation, it will prove to be profitable food for thought and open a whole world of priorities that might not otherwise have presented themselves.

David Taylor
Assistant Concertmaster, Chicago Symphony Orchestra

*Performance without Pain* provides a wealth of ideas on how to heal chronic pain and inflammation through dietary changes. This may prove an invaluable resource to musicians who battle chronic injury and have never even considered the possible impact of nutrition.

Baird Dodge
Principal Second Violin,
Chicago Symphony Orchestra

*Performance without Pain* is a remarkable book about surviving prevailing medical "wisdoms," dogmas and devastating ailments caused not by bad genes or bad lack, but by foods which are, amazingly, considered "wholesome" and "healthy." If you are a concerned parent, promising professional, aspiring artist, successful executive or simply a health-conscious and responsible individual, you must read this book to assure yourself and your children a productive and disease-free future.

Konstantin Monastyrsky
Author of *Fiber Menace*

I know that this approach to eating works, as it has, over the past five years, changed my life dramatically for the better also. You can do yourself a wonderful favor by reading this book, and trying it!

Catriona White
University Dance Professor, Former Ballet Dancer

# Performance without Pain

# Performance without Pain

A Step-by-Step Nutritional Program
for Healing Pain, Inflammation
and Chronic Ailments
in Musicians, Athletes, Dancers. . .
and Everyone Else

Kathryne Pirtle,
Clarinetist of the Orion Ensemble

with Sally Fallon,
President of the Weston A. Price Foundation

Introduction by Dr. John D. Turner, DC, CCSP, DIBCN,
former National Qualifying Gymnast

# Performance without Pain

A Step-by-Step Nutritional Program for Healing
Pain, Inflammation and Chronic Ailments
in Musicians, Athletes, Dancers. . .
and Everyone Else

Kathryne Pirtle
with Sally Fallon
Introduction by Dr. John D. Turner, DC, CCSP, DIBCN

Text font: ITC Stone Serif Standard Medium
Title font: Monotype Corsive

*Performance without Pain* is intended solely for informational and educational purposes and not as personal medical advice. Please consult your health care professional if you have any questions about your health. Testimonials regarding soy published in this book have been changed in details to protect the identity of the individuals who provided them. Neither the author nor the publisher has received financial support from the beef or dairy industries.

NewTrends Publishing, Inc.
Washington, DC    20005

www.NewTrendsPublishing.com    newtrends@kconline.com
US and Canadian Orders (877) 707-1776
Available to the trade through
Biblio Distribution (a division of NBN) (800) 462-6420

Printings: 5,000, 5,000

ISBN   0-9670897-7-8       978-0-9670897-7-5
PRINTED IN THE UNITED STATES OF AMERICA

To all people in pursuit
of their dreams and spiritual potential,
since accurate knowledge
of the nutritional requirements for human health
is essential to that end.

# CONTENTS

# ACKNOWLEDGMENTS

My gratitude and love go first to my husband Ray, my children Shelby and Morgan, and my parents Clarence and Lenore DuPree, for their unending support through my illness, my recovery and the writing of this book.

I owe an incredible debt of gratitude to my treasured friend, Dr. John Turner, for helping me in my recovery and for joining me to write this book and present lectures on this critical topic.

I am forever grateful to Sally Fallon, who has become a cherished friend through our partnership in writing and publishing. She is a beacon of light for the world through her creation of the Weston A. Price Foundation, as she guides a growing movement of people who desire a true understanding of the nutritional requirements for optimal human health, and as she helps initiate the essential return of traditional foods and farming systems.

I thank Dr. Ron Schmid and Jordan Rubin for their role in my recovery, and in helping countless people in their journey of healing.

I am indebted to my close colleagues of the Orion Ensemble—Florentina Ramniceanu, Diana Schmück, Judy Stone, Marlise Klein and Jennifer Marlas—who supported me through my illness. May our sisterhood continue to create music that inspires and lifts spirits.

Finally, I thank all the gifted individuals who helped review our book and gave it enormous support.

# PREFACE

*T*he inspiration to pursue training as a musician, dancer or athlete usually begins at a very young age in comparison with other fields. Early in their development, students learn to engage in a high level of consistent energy output and refined muscle activity. Unique to musicians are the postures they sustain while playing their instruments and the extensive repetitive use of the same muscle groups. Because of these factors, most people in these fields experience injuries and, often, chronic pain.

Repetitive-use injuries are some of the most common problems to afflict musicians, dancers and athletes—and even those engaged in more mundane activities, such as using the computer or operating machine tools. These injuries can be extremely frightening, especially to the professional performer, for many reasons. First is the uncertainty of not knowing which course of action to take when you are feeling pain. The pain may be quite debilitating both physically and mentally and cause the artist or athlete to work with great discomfort;

even worse, the injury may make performance impossible, even if the pain affects only one small area. If we continue to "work through the pain," the injury may become more serious. An untreated or inappropriately treated injury may threaten our career potential. Unfortunately, we may have to do extensive research to find the best treatment, which may involve coordinating many types of approaches for the complete resolution of the problem. If we do not undertake a thorough investigation of all the possible factors that may have caused the injury, similar problems are certain to plague us in the future.

Some of the most prevalent types of injuries are inflammatory—such as tendonitis, overuse disorders and trauma to the hands or upper and lower extremities—and muscle strength impairment. The traditional approach to treating inflammatory injuries of performing artists and athletes usually involves extensive physical therapy, often including the use of anti-inflammatory medication. For muscle weakness, combining adequate rest periods with careful attention to technique is often helpful. The artist or athlete can also work with private teachers, trainers or body-use specialists to refine his or her movements so that they require less effort, adopting a regimen that balances the muscles of the body to help prevent future injury. These are well-documented treatments and sometimes provide relief from the injury.

However, when injuries continue, even after thoughtful application of these approaches, other underlying causes must be considered. An artist or athlete may actually be predisposed to injuries because of certain dietary factors such as inadequate nutrition, a pro-inflammatory diet, food allergies, digestive disorders and malabsorption.

As a professional clarinetist, I suffered recurring serious inflammations during my twenties and thirties. These affected my playing, and through the treatments I pursued at that time, they did go away. I received regular chiropractic care, saw a massage therapist, developed stretching and strengthening routines, applied the principles of the Alexander technique, and tried to eat a very "good" diet by following modern nutritional dictates and the USDA Food Pyramid. However, my symptoms often recurred, though their intensity was not debilitating, for I had learned many physical-therapy treatments that were effective in controlling them. In retrospect, the symptoms I had were actually signs of a very serious undiagnosed allergy to gluten-containing grains (such as wheat, rye, and barley) called celiac disease, which causes a digestive disorder.

In my forties I developed another, far more severe inflammation in my spine along with embouchure shaking, and I became gravely ill with malabsorption. (The embouchure involves muscles around the mouth used to play wind instruments.) This debilitating condition nearly ended my well-established career. When I finally was diagnosed with gluten sensitivity, I had already incurred the long-term effects of celiac disease—extensive malnourishment from malabsorption and intestinal damage. Through intensive research, I found the solutions to my life-long nutritional deficits in the work of a scientist who studied the diets of healthy isolated cultures worldwide—Dr. Weston Price. The principles of a healthy diet that he formulated almost completely contradict the lowfat, high-carb dictates of our modern medical institutions. I came to realize that my problems were similar to the many degenerative conditions experienced by others in our society and were the result of drastic changes to our food supply beginning in the early 1900s. The answer for me was very complex and could not be remedied by the standard treatments in our field. Rather, it involved a radical change in my diet.

Thus, I am suggesting that even though you believe your diet to be perfect, and even though your injuries go away with common types of treatments, the fact that you were injured in the first place may indicate that you need to take a careful look at your nutrition. Many factors in the modern diet can predispose you to inflammation and inadequate muscle energy. Your tendency towards injury and inflammation may also be a precursor to a more serious chronic ailment later in your life.

Musicians, athletes and dancers require extremely high levels of repetitive muscle and tendon use but, in terms of the body's physiological priority, maintenance of muscles and tendons is not at the top of the list. The body expends energy and nutrients on other systems—the brain, the organs and digestion—before the muscles and tendons receive their allocation. When we experience recurring injuries, we must carefully consider the possibility that dietary deficiencies as well as other more serious health issues may be causing a predisposition to injury, lack of stamina and inadequate resources to focus repair energy on muscles and tendons.

Artists and athletes should also keep in mind that even when they have no injuries, they can benefit from superior nutrition. If we expect to have vibrant longevity in our demanding fields, we cannot separate this objective from the need to be well nourished. We need to consider the possible long-term positive or negative effects of the foods we choose to eat. We can only enhance our performance (including our concentration skills) when we make dietary choices that support our overall physical well-being.

In this book we will examine the dietary elements that may influence overall health and a predisposition to injury, inflammatory conditions and muscle strength impairment. We will discuss how nutrition can affect the body's ability to maintain and repair itself. In the area of food quality, we will examine the changes in the way our foods have been produced and how this has drastically affected the health of many people. Finally, we will present a practical plan for obtaining foods that can adequately support our need for superior nutrition.

Sally Fallon, author, international lecturer and founding president of the Weston Price Foundation, joins me as a co-author of this book. Her input will help you find nutritional answers to injury prevention, and to the relief of pain, inflammation and chronic ailments with an approach that unites the dietary wisdom of primitive cultures—which were immune to disease and degenerative conditions—and the latest independent and accurate scientific research. Sally's renowned book, *Nourishing Traditions,* helped me to pull together the sometimes contradictory strands of information that I had discovered throughout the years of my research. Through our collaboration, we bring you a concise resource that can help you achieve vibrant health and help keep you pain and injury free.

The need for this book became clear in 2004 when I contacted Nick Quarrier, the clinical associate professor of physical therapy in charge of an injury-prevention workshop at Ithaca College in New York. I saw that the topics covered in their workshop did not include nutrition and wanted to speak at the conference about my experience. I contacted Nick and told him my story. He was astounded at the timing of my call, as his sister, who is a triathlon athlete, had just been diagnosed with gluten sensitivity and had many problems with inflammation. He asked me to write a paper about my experience for the conference. Just as he received my manuscript, he had an appointment with a young violist in her twenties whose problems with rheumatoid arthritis made playing very difficult. She also had allergies to wheat. He shared my paper with her to give her insight into the possible relationship of her diet to her illness. Nick also told me about a classical guitarist he knew who had suffered for years from the same types of problems I had experienced. He said, "She is just like you!"

Unfortunately, accurate principles of good nutrition are not yet common knowledge, and few recognize the dangers of modern dietary habits. In fact, I looked at all the published research on musicians' injuries since 1980 and found no studies linking poor nutrition with a predisposition to injury. Yet I had become increasingly convinced that my predisposition was *definitely* caused by nutritional factors stemming from changes to our food supply over the last 60 years. I also recognized the fact that many others who had suffered from the same problems had not found satisfying answers.

When I presented my paper at the conference in June 2004, many artists who attended recognized my symptoms in themselves. Nick Quarrier told me that this information was the missing link in his practice, and that it was essential that I write a book to engage artists in a new understanding about the nutritional factors in injuries.

Thus, with the encouragement of Nick Quarrier and Sally Fallon, I began writing in June of 2004 with the hope that the principles in this book will help musicians, athletes and many others understand the integral relationship of a carefully chosen diet with the prevention of injury and overall good health.

Subsequently, in the fall of 2004, John D. Turner, DC, CCSP, DIBCN and I began to present lectures at universities on the relationship of nutrition to injuries for music students. Dr. Turner, a prominent chiropractic physician in the Chicago area who has worked with musicians, dancers and elite athletes, had played a key role in helping me recover from my illness. He is a board certified chiropractic neurologist and is also certified in acupuncture and sports medicine. In our seminars, we have found that many of the musicians present had symptoms of digestion problems and had experienced recurring inflammatory tendencies along with muscle weakness and embouchure instability. We have also seen many vocalists who are struggling with acid-reflux disease, a serious condition that can affect the vocal cords. In addition, we have been asked to speak in schools and in community lecture series about critical health and nutrition issues as they relate to our food supply.

The information in this book is not for musicians, athletes and dancers alone, but also for the general public. With the looming health implications of our degraded food supply, and digestive and related chronic illnesses affecting an escalating percentage of our population, more and more people are finding answers to healing through the invaluable principles found in this approach. As we prepared a book geared toward the health of artists and athletes, and as Dr. Turner and I began speaking to a wide range of audiences, it became clear that this concise guide could serve as a practical resource for anyone wishing to achieve better health.

Kathryne Pirtle
January, 2006

# INTRODUCTION

*T*he tragic irony of our decline in national health is the fact that it is happening right before our eyes and with our consent! Despite the overwhelming evidence that we are needlessly suffering from arthritis, heart disease, diabetes, hypertension and many other debilitating diseases, we continue to consume the refined and chemically laced "food" that is contributing to these horrible conditions. After twenty years of assisting patients return to health, I have often concluded that it is easier to get someone to quit smoking than it is to get them to change their diets. Besides the emotional factors that accompany eating, specific biochemical factors draw us to certain foods. This is no secret to the profit-oriented food industry that supplies the majority of us with our meals. There is hope, however. Books like this and Sally Fallon's *Nourishing Traditions* are creating a groundswell that is growing in power because the authors are revealing the truth about our diet and how it influences our health.

We are all exposed to parasites, toxins, viruses and unfriendly bacteria on a daily basis. Why is it that some people escape the invasion while others do not? The gastrointestinal tract is our first line of defense against these hostile invaders. The condition of the mucosal lining of the intestines should therefore be a top priority in our quest for optimal health. The proper fats, probiotic colonization, nutrients and enzymes are supplied by the traditional foods discussed in this book. These foods will create an impenetrable wall of defense in our intestines.

Consider the intestinal wall as a filtering mechanism, similar to a membrane air filter that sits in the furnace of your home. The gut wall is comprised of "villi" or folds, which if flattened out, would have the surface area equal to that of a football field! That vast surface is needed to absorb nutrients into our bloodstream once they have been extracted from the food we eat. An air filter whose membrane has large gaps and holes will allow dust particles and pollens to pass through. Likewise, a gut wall that has large gaps and areas of poor integrity will allow complex food particles, pollens and parasites to pass through when they would normally be filtered out. This condition is called "leaky gut." The consequences of a leaky gut are the common health problems with which most of us are familiar—food allergies, irritable bowel syndrome, chronic fatigue, intestinal cramping, bloating and gas.

The integrity of our intestines is highly dependent on the quality and types of foods and fats we eat. As a modern society, we are severely depleted in nutrients and quality fats (including saturated fats) and suffer from imbalances in the fatty acid ratios in our diets due to our consumption of harmful industrially processed fats and oils.

Because of the nutritional and structural imbalances that are a direct result of what we eat, our ability to meet the demands of a rigorous and hectic life can be severely compromised. This is especially true for professional musicians, athletes and dancers who juggle performances or games, practice, family, personal life and, sometimes, another job. They are required to undergo strenuous, repetitive and highly focused activities, and to not make any mistakes. Their bodies, therefore, require an optimal physical and nutritional status to perform injury-free at top levels.

The impetus for this book came from my experience with the author, Kathy Pirtle, who was going through career-ending health challenges several years ago. Kathy had spent years perfecting her skills as a musician and had achieved a level of performance that placed her at the top of her field. She began to suffer from severe neck, shoulder and arm pain both during and away from her performances. After a lack of results with conventional methods, Kathy turned to alternative techniques and eventually ended up in my office. We were able to relieve her symptoms with chiropractic treatments, but only temporarily. It wasn't until we began to correct nutritional deficiencies and address the digestion-related repercussions of an underlying gluten sensitivity that a deeper, more permanent healing could occur.

Another dramatic example in my practice that demonstrated the interrelationship between inflammation and an ailment of the digestive system occurred in a woman with a bowel-induced musculoskeletal disorder. She was in her late forties and had been suffering from migrating polyarthralgias for over five years. Each day she would awaken to pain and swelling in a different joint in her body. One day a finger would be swollen and red, the next day it might be a knee or shoulder. No pattern emerged, and conventional medicine had failed to reveal the source of her malady. This fact was significant in that she worked at a large hospital and had access to the latest and greatest that modern medicine could offer.

Knowing this, I decided to investigate the one area that had gone unnoticed—her intestinal tract. Laboratory results revealed an abundance of a pathogenic bacterium. After some research I discovered that this "wee beastie" secretes an endotoxin that can be absorbed through the wall of the intestines and that finds its way into the synovial fluid of the joints, causing arthritis-like symptoms! Who would have thought that such a link existed? We started on a course of healing that involved nutritional and homeopathic supplements, herbs and dietary changes. She was soon pain free and moving on with her life.

As a chiropractic physician, I see the consequences of inflammation on a daily basis. Inflammation is at the heart of most of our chronic pains. Pain registers in the brain because an inflammatory chemical somewhere in the body stimulates a nerve. The location, quality and intensity of the pain are all registered by different parts of the brain. It is a very complex system, but the important point is that it is a chemically driven process.

Why is it that two patients with identical injuries can experience entirely different levels of pain? Although the two injuries may be *biomechanically* the same, the two patients are *biochemically* different! That means the same injury will cause debilitating pain in one person and only a mild discomfort in another. There can also be genetic factors at work, but the most influential factor is the amount of inflammation already present in each person. Food allergies, consumption of food additives and nutritional status all contribute to the amount of inflammation, and therefore pain, in our bodies at any given time.

Another cause of increased pain is the accumulation of chemicals that manufacturers add to our foods to enhance flavor, color and shelf life and also the chemicals that are produced by our bodies as a consequence of ingesting allergenic and denatured foods. Chemical irritants like histamine, 5-hydroxytryptamine, leukotriene B-4, bradykinins and prostaglandin E-2 are produced by our bodies and can "pre-load" the receptor sites of the nerves, which in turn transmit pain signals to our brains. That means it takes less *real* neurotransmitter substance to stimulate the nerve and therefore "feel" the pain.

Despite the work of Dr. Weston Price in the 1930s, which documented the benefits of traditional foods and diets, modern medicine has only recently admitted the fact that diet has anything to do with health; worse, the dietary advice it proffers is filled with misinformation. Today's politically correct lowfat, high-grain dietary paradigm is actually a recipe for inflammatory conditions and pain.

Modern medicine has a *disease*-oriented approach to health. Most doctors in the United States have been trained to look at *health* as merely the absence of symptoms. I actually had a patient report that her medical doctor told her to come back when her symptoms were worse because she was not sick enough to diagnose! Physicians in traditional societies look at health as optimal vitality, a vitality that comes from the foods we consume and that manifests as an engagement in mental, physical and spiritual activity on a consistent basis. I have heard that in some "less evolved" countries, a patient will fire his doctor if he becomes sick too often, because the doctor's job is to keep them well!

We have become a society looking for a quick solution to our health problems—most of which are a direct result of the food we are eating. Think of all the television ads for products to treat stomach pain, bloating, gas, acid reflux, indigestion, constipation, diarrhea and heartburn. These are all symptoms of an imbalance in the gastrointestinal tract and they are *not* due to a deficiency of the products being sold on television!

They can, however, be due to nutritional deficiencies and imbalances created by our modern diets and the diets of our parents. Today's products and drugs used to treat digestive complaints merely mask the symptoms; they do not solve the problem. Only through correcting our nutrition will true healing occur.

Nutrition has always been an important part of my practice. Through years of experience working with chronic illnesses and by utilizing homeopathic, herbal and nutritional remedies that assist the body's inherent ability to detoxify, fight infections and heal, I have been able to guide patients back to healthier bodies and lifestyles. Unfortunately, this is often an uphill battle. Re-educating patients about the benefits of animal fats in their diets, repositioning grains to the top and not the base of the Food Pyramid, and motivating patients to take the time to prepare whole foods that are rich in nutrients can be very challenging. The FDA guidelines are influenced by the food industry and are not based on fact. Because it is a powerful agency, people tend not to question its recommendations.

The first step in improving your health is to take responsibility for it. No one knows your body better than you do. Do not blindly follow the masses on their way to the next fast food trend or the next lowfat vegetarian food. Realize that the majority of the food manufacturers today are in business to turn a profit and not to supply you and your family with nutritious, balanced diets. Embrace a proactive approach, which you can do by following the steps outlined in this book and taking the time to prepare whole foods, using traditional methods. Above all, do not be afraid of animal fats (the best coming from traditionally raised animals)—they are *vital* to good health. The plan outlined here will start you on a path of recovery towards your natural state, which is *health*, not disease.

John D. Turner, DC, CCSP, DIBCN
January, 2006

# 1

# MY STORY

## *"You can't play an instrument without your body!"*

*I* am a professional musician, the clarinetist and executive director of the Orion Ensemble, founded in 1992. We tour throughout North America, present three series each year in the Chicago metropolitan area, and perform a live, internationally broadcast series on WFMT, Fine Arts Radio in Chicago. I am also Principal Clarinetist of the Lake Forest Symphony and frequently perform with the Lyric Opera, the Grant Park Symphony, the Ravinia Festival Orchestra and the Chicago Symphony. In addition, I have served on the faculties of the Wheaton College Conservatory of Music, Northern Illinois University, Indiana University and Bradley University.

In 2004, the Hal Leonard Corporation released my solo album of selected Bach unaccompanied cello and violin suites and sonatas transcribed for the clarinet by Himie Voxman. This represents the first time these transcriptions have been presented in a recording by a clarinetist.

# Performance without Pain

My passion for my work has been boundless since the age of six, when I became inspired to become a musician. However, because of inflammatory conditions throughout my training and career, playing my instrument often entailed a great deal of pain and suffering. In my early twenties, whenever I practiced for long periods, I regularly experienced pain and numbness in my shoulders, arms and fingers. This would come and go depending on my repertoire and performance schedule. I never thought much about these symptoms because they would "go away." At age twenty-five, I developed TMJ syndrome, a painful inflammation that prevented me from opening my mouth—definitely an impediment for a clarinet player! I looked at more efficient ways to use my embouchure—the crucial facial muscles that wind players use to produce a beautiful sound—and began using a mouth guard at night to prevent my jaw muscles from clenching and the consequent inflammation.

It was during my late twenties, when I was playing in the Chicago Civic Orchestra, that my symptoms began to frighten me. My neck and back started to hurt, and my arms, hands and fingers had numbness and shooting pain. I had to quit playing for about a month, finding only temporary relief from my symptoms through measures recommended by medical doctors familiar with musicians' problems.

During this time, I was in the midst of auditions. Before the Milwaukee Symphony principal clarinet audition, I had to lie on ice cubes for relief from intense pain in my upper back. Luckily, I started working with a good chiropractor. I also studied the Alexander technique, began regular massage therapy, used ice to help prevent and treat any inflammation, and supported my instrument with an ergonomic neck strap while resting the bell of the clarinet on my legs. These therapies helped to heal my body and became my prescription for taking care of myself and dealing with pain in my neck, shoulders and arms.

In my mid-thirties my career began to develop in many exciting ways. Besides orchestral work and teaching, I helped found the Orion Ensemble. However, I was plagued with a feeling of stiffness in my arms and back. I did not want to ignore this new symptom for fear of more serious complications. I found that by adding a regular yoga routine paired with muscle-balancing exercises to my daily fitness regimen, I was much more limber. I literally became an expert on body-use and body-balancing techniques and the benefits of chiropractic care and massage therapy. I thought I could handle any pain!

I should also point out that I became deeply interested in nutrition at this time and sought answers to the question, "What is the most nutritious diet that I can follow?" I embraced the popular guidelines for healthy eating based on the principles of the USDA Food Pyramid: lots of salads, whole wheat bread, vegetables and fruits, along with some meat, chicken, eggs and dairy. I bought mostly organic foods at the health food store. I also took a carefully chosen array of vitamin and mineral supplements, including a whole food supplement called "Super Blue-Green Algae," which was touted as the greatest super-food known to man! My only vices were a few cookies and one cup of coffee a day. I wanted to be as healthy as possible, to feel my best and keep up with the physical demands of performance.

When I was forty-two, I realized I was developing acid reflux disease, a condition in which stomach acid is released up through the esophagus, causing damage to the esophageal lining. I constantly felt the need to burp, which resulted in the horrible feel and taste of stomach acid rising into my throat. This, I later discovered, was also a symptom of a developing hiatal hernia. With observation and personal experimentation I discovered that if I didn't eat wheat, my symptoms would go away. I began following the principles of the "blood-type diet," which for me, a type-O, meant eating more meat, fish, vegetables and fruit; drinking herbal and green teas instead of coffee; and switching from wheat to rice, rye crackers and wheat-free cookies—it was worth the sacrifice to feel better. I had made so many changes over the years to be "healthy," I could certainly do this!

My new diet gave me some relief, but it was no cure. By age forty-five, my right arm and shoulder were hurting all the time. No matter what I did—chiropractic, massage therapy, stretching—all of the things

I knew—the discomfort was constant. During the next few months I developed an inflammation in my spine that made it very difficult and painful to use my hands and fingers. If I used my arms to carry my compact clarinet case, lift a load of laundry or wash the floor, I experienced an increase in pain intensity for several days. At the time, I was playing in the backstage orchestra with the Lyric Opera of Chicago and preparing for five performances of the Brahms Quintet plus a multitude of other important concerts. My pain horrified me. What would the answer be this time—or would there be an answer? Would my career be over? I was at the height of my profession—I had worked for so many years—and I didn't want to do anything else.

My chiropractor, Dr. John Turner, helped me to find the source of this inflammatory condition as well as the key to what had happened in years past. His diagnosis: an allergy or sensitivity to gluten called celiac disease. This disease often goes undiagnosed for many years until the symptoms become quite serious. With this sensitivity, gluten, a protein found in wheat, rye and barley, causes intestinal damage, which leads to digestive malabsorption and eventually severe malnourishment. A mere *microgram* of gluten can cause intestinal damage in people with celiac disease. When my pain reached its peak, I was eating only one or two rye crackers a day and no wheat at all. However, this dietary practice followed a lifetime of gluten consumption. I learned that gluten sensitivity is becoming extremely common, along with digestion and malabsorption problems.

My next self-imposed discipline was complete avoidance of foods containing gluten. This, by the way, is no easy task, as many foods you would never suspect contain gluten, even drinks such as herbal teas and coffee substitutes with "roasted barley malt." I studied the celiac disease list of "foods that contain gluten" with a fine-tooth comb so that I would not accidentally ingest even a microgram of the forbidden substance. Eating out posed unique challenges! At the same time, I gave up all sugar. After avoiding gluten and sugar completely for two weeks, I began to experience an unusual burning sensation on my skin from the top of my head all the way down to my toes, along with a feeling of nausea. This lasted for about three weeks. I learned that these sensations were a sign of detoxification. Although frightened, I accepted this as evidence that my body was going through a profound healing process. When you have an allergy or sensitivity to a food, you actually crave that food, and its use causes a drug-like addiction. The burning sensations were a sign of a drug withdrawal.

After following a gluten-free and sugar-free diet for about a month, all the inflammatory symptoms in my spine disappeared. The summer was wonderful! I was pain-free for the first time in a year, and my practicing gave me great joy.

However, when my teaching and my performing schedule began in the fall, a new problem appeared: diarrhea. I was going to the bathroom about six or seven times a day, losing weight steadily, unable to sleep and feeling quite weak. More frightening was the fact that my embouchure was shaking uncontrollably. I could not even play one line of music without feeling that my sound was out of control. I was preparing to perform the Hindemith Quartet in our chamber music series and on WFMT Fine Arts Radio. The Hindemith Quartet requires more endurance than almost any other piece in our repertoire. I also had a challenging week playing with the orchestra. What in the world could be wrong with me now? I had been eating a completely nutritious diet. Why was I still so sick?

My chiropractor explained that my allergy had been causing intestinal damage for many years and that I had a long-term problem with malabsorption and its related malnourishment—that, even though I was eating a superb diet, it would take significant time for the digestive track to heal. I was literally *starving*. In terms of traditional acupuncture, embouchure shaking relates to the "digestion meridian" in the body. Because I was still in a very depleted state, the stability of my embouchure was affected. My insomnia was also related to my digestion problem. My doctor prescribed a new supplement with concentrated nutrition made from fish protein, which could be absorbed through the blood stream and could help heal my intestinal lining. This supplement, although very nutritious, was not enough to change my symptoms as quickly as I needed. I sought more information to correct my digestive disorder.

It was at this point in my odyssey that I discovered the work of Jordan Rubin, who nearly died and then recovered from a severe digestive disorder called Crohn's disease. The pianist in our chamber group, Diana Schmück, gave me his book, *Patient Heal Thyself,* which describes his descent into malnutrition hell, an experience that mirrored my own, including my frequent trips to the bathroom! I followed his plan for improving digestion. I started taking a green-food supplement, which offered an easy-to-digest source of concentrated nutrition. I began a superior powdered enzyme supplement, which helped my digestive system break down the foods that I was eating. I added a soil-based organism supplement (SBO), as well as coconut oil, which helped me develop a healthy intestinal bacterial flora. I also added cod liver oil, which supplies the fats necessary for the proper digestion of foods and the fat-soluble nutrients needed for the assimilation of nutrients. Using Jordan's protocol, I soon felt improvement. I stopped going to the bathroom so many times, and my embouchure gradually regained stability. Jordan's work helped me define the first principle of my recovery: establishing a healthy digestive ecosystem.

The second principle involves easy-to-digest foods that provide the gut with the nutrients it needs to heal. . . unfortunately the diet I considered so healthy was not providing these foods. My introduction to these foods came through the work of Dr. Weston Price, DDS, and his book *Nutrition and Physical Degeneration*. During the 1930s, Price traveled worldwide and carefully studied fourteen healthy isolated populations untouched by modern civilization, from isolated Swiss and Irish to Eskimos, Peruvian Indians and Africans. While their diets differed in exact details, all contained distinct common characteristics which, without exception, had given them vibrant health from generation to generation. Price analyzed their foods and found that they were very rich in vitamins and minerals and extremely rich in two specific vitamins: A and D. Price developed a therapy involving a combination of high-vitamin cod liver oil and high-vitamin butter oil, which he found miraculously effective for healing the tendons, muscles, nerves. . . and the gut.

I then applied Price's principles of a nutrient-dense diet by obtaining naturally raised meats, eggs, raw dairy and poultry from a cooperative of farmers dedicated to raising their animals on pasture. (Pasture-raising maximizes the nutrients in our food, especially the fat-soluble vitamins like A and D in the animal fats.) I began, for the first time in my life, to drink clean raw milk (made into a fermented drink called kefir) and to experience raw cream, cheese and butter—all traditional foods that had nourished healthy populations for thousands of years, but ones we now mostly avoid due to the mistaken notion that these high-fat foods are bad for us. I began the high-vitamin cod liver oil and high-vitamin butter oil therapy. I also learned traditional techniques of preserving food through lacto-fermentation, a process that was used universally before refrigeration and is still practiced in nonindustrialized cultures. I prepared lacto-fermented foods such as sauerkraut and a medicinal drink called beet kvass from traditional recipes. They provided enzymes, beneficial bacteria, lactic acid and many nutrients in easily assimilated form, all of which benefit the digestive tract. These extremely nutritious foods and supplements became the backbone of my healing regimen.

By the time of my Hindemith performances, I was well enough to play. I gradually put on the weight that I had lost, was able to get restful sleep at night, and could tell that my body was beginning to absorb more of the incredible nutrients in my diet. There is an old saying: *"It's not what you eat, it's what you absorb."* I truly learned that truth first hand. How many years had my body been unable to absorb the nutrients in the foods I was eating? I suspect it may have been my entire life!

Even though I was much better, I still experienced some symptoms of long-term malnourishment. I was preparing to play a sonata in our series and was doing about 15 minutes of practicing while standing every day—I generally play orchestral and chamber music in a seated position. After my second month of preparation, I experienced quite a bit of pain in my right shoulder. Apparently, even though I had used a neckstrap, the pressure from pushing my instrument forward in a standing position without the benefit of leg support caused a soft tissue injury in my shoulder due to my body's still depleted condition. Then, in trying to stretch the tight muscles in that area, I actually sprained my neck! Just to be sure I didn't have a disc problem in my neck, I underwent testing and was relieved to learn that my cervical vertebrae had excellent spacing. But this very painful sprain and soft tissue injury took about six months to heal.

This injury convinced me that I should fine-tune my dietary approach by seeking consultation with a doctor who specialized in treating chronic illness with a traditional diet. I began to work with Dr. Ron Schmid, a naturopathic physician from Connecticut, who had 25 years of experience in treating chronic illness through traditional foods and the principles of Dr. Weston Price. Dr. Schmid had recovered from a serious digestive disorder many years earlier, and his recovery inspired him to become a naturopathic physician. With the aid of a special blood test to help determine my health status, he was able to help recommend a few additional dietary measures that enabled my final recovery. Under Dr. Schmid's care, I continued the primitive diet that I had already developed from my own research, but with some changes: I significantly increased the amount of clean raw milk kefir from pastured cows in place of fruit or nut snacks; added homemade gelatin-rich bone broths to my diet; eliminated even gluten-free grains such as rice from my diet; doubled my dose of cod-liver oil and high-vitamin butter oil; began special vitamin E and vitamin C supplements, plus additive-free calcium/magnesium, a multivitamin and milk thistle supplements that Dr. Schmid developed; and took two other supplements to help build my depleted adrenal glands.

My new, easier-to-digest traditional diet also had another important feature—it was low in fiber! The few vegetables that I now consumed were cooked in bone-broth soup, steamed and served with butter or lacto-fermented, and the foods that I added were nutrient-dense foods that contained no fiber. Since my recovery, I have learned from

# 1. My Story

a book called *Fiber Menace,* by Konstantin Monastyrsky, that modern high-fiber diets—although thought to be healthy—can wreak havoc on the digestive system. This is largely due to the fact that these diets are not only low in nutrient-density, but also because they do not provide the critical dietary components necessary for nutrient absorption and proper digestive function. Traditional healthy diets that included fiber from grains and vegetables also supplied adequate fats, vitamins A and D, easy-to-digest bone broth soups, lacto-fermented foods that promote a healthy intestinal flora and high-quality sources of protein. Healthy cultures, however, ate very few raw vegetables and fruits because they were consumed only in season. Additionally, many of the cultures that Dr. Price studied ate very little fiber at all.

Mr. Monastyrsky, a brilliant man who suffered and recovered from a life-threatening illness that he developed during his years as a vegetarian, has written two best-selling Russian language books, *Functional Nutrition: The Foundation of Absolute Health and Longevity,* and *Disorders of Carbohydrate Metabolism.* He reveals the disastrous effects our modern high-fiber nutritional dictates can have on the proper functioning of the digestive system. From large stools—which stretch the intestinal tract beyond its normal range and eventually cause intestinal damage and bowel problems, including hernias, hemorrhoidal disease, constipation, malnourishment, irritable bowel syndrome and Crohn's disease—to a drastic upset of the natural bacterial flora in the intestinal tract, *Fiber Menace* describes major health issues that can develop from eating what's considered a modern "healthy" diet high in fiber from grains, vegetables, fruits and legumes and even fiber supplements.

From years of following the Food Pyramid—eating lots of hard-to-digest raw vegetables and grains that are also low in nutrient density, avoiding traditional fats and protein, and remaining unaware of the importance of lacto-fermented foods—I had wiped out the healthy bacteria and mucosa in my gut. This damage, coupled with the damage wrought by celiac disease, had severely compromised nutrient absorption. Several years later, I learned that my hiatal hernia could have been caused from the constant fermentation of all these hard-to-digest foods. It seems hard to believe that just two generations before I was born, my sturdy ancestors had, for hundreds of generations, enjoyed traditional farm diets loaded with fats, high-quality proteins and foods that preserved the integrity of the digestive system. Salads were not even in their cuisine. My modern "healthy diet" had been so far from healthy!

Within two weeks of implementing these additional measures, I was totally pain free and felt a heightened sense of well-being. It was so exciting to feel well! I knew these additional details were the missing elements in my path to optimal health.

Dr. Schmid explained that my embouchure-shaking symptom was very serious. Had I not taken the steps to heal this problem, I could have become gravely ill.

It took well over a year and a half to recover completely, and I continue to notice improvements in my health. I now follow a gluten-free, nutrient dense, high-enzyme diet that includes an abundance of foods to maintain the healthy bacterial flora in my digestive track. I make sure that I consume optimal amounts of vitamins A and D and include a wide variety of specific, high-quality unprocessed fats and oils that promote good digestion and assimilation, cell building, repair and a healthy nervous system. In addition, I include bone-broth soups in my diet daily and eat meat, poultry, dairy and eggs from traditionally raised pasture-fed animals. I eat absolutely no refined foods of any kind.

My lifetime passion spent as an artist and teacher is far too precious to lose. My goal is to continue performing for many years to come. But I can't play music without my body! I am grateful to be playing my instrument, performing and enjoying life—pain-free!

## 2

# ESTABLISHING
# A HEALTHY ECOSYSTEM

*E*stablishing a healthy intestinal ecosystem is of prime importance in obtaining the maximum benefit of nutrition from the foods you eat. A healthy intestinal ecosystem also contributes to a strong immune system. It is the first principle for regaining and maintaining good health.

Today, many people, including young people, experience digestive problems, which eventually lead to malabsorption, malnourishment and a weakened immune system because their digestive tracts lack the ability to thoroughly break down food. This is due to intestinal damage caused by the ongoing incomplete digestion of foods stemming from inadequate healthy intestinal bacterial flora. Since the influx of refined foods, refrigeration, antibiotics and chlorinated water, people have become more susceptible to bacterial imbalance and fermentation in the gut.

Developing beneficial bacteria in the gut is the first step to overcoming digestion and absorption issues. Only when the gut has a healthy ecosystem can the healing process of your muscles, tendons and other body systems begin. Musicians understand what happens when they practice incorrectly—nothing positive and lasting. For all of us, working on digestion is like practicing correctly—it is the basis for fixing the problem.

When most people think of bacteria, they think of something that makes us sick—something undesirable. However, in your intestinal tract live one hundred trillion bacteria and other microorganisms—more bacterial cells than anywhere else in your body. The friendly bacteria in your gut—called your intestinal flora—keep harmful bacteria like salmonella, fungus like *Candida albicans*, parasites and other disease-causing microorganisms in check, preventing them from attaching themselves to the walls of your intestinal tract where they can cause real damage. Good bacteria also help the body ward off abnormal cells, such as cancer cells, and toxic substances. When in proper balance, these beneficial bacteria and microbes promote health and well-being—they strengthen your immune system and help break down your food into its usable components so that valuable nutrients can be absorbed. The proper functioning of the entire body depends on optimal digestion.

The modern diet presents many challenges to maintaining a healthy intestinal flora. Drastic changes to our food supply have caused a dramatic increase in the prevalence of digestion problems. Most people are consuming large amounts of refined foods that remain undigested in the colon and can cause an overgrowth of bad bacteria. Furthermore, we are guilty of an enormous overuse of antibiotics, which destroy the good bacteria along with the bad, leaving room for antibiotic-resistant bacteria, yeast and fungi to grow in the gut, and the pervasive use of antacids and acid-blocking medications neutralize hydrochloric acid in the stomach, allowing harmful bacteria to pass into the intestines.

Chlorinated water, now in most homes, kills both the helpful and harmful bacteria in the gut.

Finally, since the dawn of refrigeration, people no longer con-

# 2. Establishing a Healthy EcoSystem

sume fermented foods such as sauerkraut, pickles, kefir and yogurt, naturally preserved by a process called lacto-fermentation, which greatly increases the levels of friendly bacteria in our food.

The best way to begin changing your inner body ecology is to eat foods that are whole, unrefined, high in nutrients and easy to digest. Instead of refined grains and sugar, which clearly support harmful intestinal bacteria, choose high-quality meats, organ meats, poultry, eggs and raw dairy, preferably from pastured animals. Soups made from bone broths are also enormously nutritious and easy to digest (more on bone broths later). Choose a variety of wild-caught fish and seafood. Focus carbohydrate consumption on vegetables, limit fruit and avoid fruit juice. (A low-carbohydrate diet helps to "starve" the bad bacteria.) Eat plenty of high-quality fats such as butter and coconut oil, which support digestion and encourage good bacteria.

Next, it is critical to consume foods and beverages that enhance the good bacteria in your intestinal system and to consume them everyday. These lacto-fermented foods and beverages are easy to prepare (see Chapter 9). Historically, people consumed many foods and beverages preserved by lacto-fermentation. The traditional process of fermenting cow's and goat's milk into yogurt or kefir, cucumbers into pickles, cabbage into sauerkraut and kimchi, beets into beet kvass and pickled beets and countless other foods into lacto-fermented condiments and beverages from around the world, provided people's digestive systems with probiotics from the lactobacillus bacteria family. These lactic-acid-producing bacteria help create healthy flora in the gut and support enzyme function, making proteins, minerals and other nutrients more bioavailable. They also inhibit many kinds of harmful bacteria and viruses while strengthening the immune system.

Another method of enhancing bacterial flora, especially at the beginning, is to take effective probiotic supplements. Most commercial supplements are not viable as their probiotic activity is very low. The most hardy probiotic supplements come from soil-based organisms, or SBOs. In times past, our ancestors consumed soil along with their fruits and vegetables. This soil contained beneficial microorganisms necessary for optimal digestion. In our hygiene-conscious society, we scoff at the idea of having any dirt on our food—when in fact, without a little dirt, we are depriving our guts of important bacteria. SBOs (see Sources) are resilient probiotics that help to colonize a wide array of good bacteria on the walls of the intestines and displace the harmful bacteria where they have lodged. They also clean decay from the intestinal walls to optimize the absorption of nutrients.

Healthy digestive and immune systems allow the body to devote energy toward healing all body systems and to the repair and maintenance of muscles and tendons. A nutritional approach takes time, but perseverance will establish enduring health rewards.

# 3
# NUTRIENT-DENSE FOOD

*T*he second healing principle involves the consumption of nutrient-dense foods. But what are nutrient-dense foods?

Almost every day we hear a report telling us that some food is either good or bad for us. Something that was good for you last week may be reported to be bad for you in the next. There are countless weight-loss and health-promoting diets, all touted as providing the definitive solution. Even more confusing is the fact that all of these suggestions are supposedly based on scientific research. If you are 30 years old or older, you can probably list a large number of dietary trends that you have lived through, many of which are totally contradictory.

The problem with these trends is that they are just that—trends. They are not based on studies of healthy populations worldwide, populations that thrived for thousands of years, free of degenerative conditions. Our dietary trends are largely based on research that is funded by, and is for the benefit of, the industrial farming industry—a system that has totally altered the quality and kinds of foods we have available. In our industrialized society, what we have to show for our dietary choices is chronic illness that has reached epic proportions—chronic illness and degenerative conditions that are not only affecting the old, but are afflicting young people in the prime of their lives.

We all must consider the fact that our health literally will determine whether we will be able to enjoy full lives and careers. For artists and athletes, our health determines whether we can continue to pursue and enjoy our high level of performance—or be cut short, perhaps long before we are ready to retire. The search for nutrition that truly supports the human body in all its intricacies cannot be approached by looking only at trends, but by seeking out accurate information based on the dietary patterns of people who have been healthy, generation after generation—those who had no degenerative conditions such as arthritis, cancer, digestive disorders, kidney disease and so forth.

It was Dr. Weston Price who discovered the timeless principles for nourishing the human body. A prominent dentist in the 1920s, 30s and 40s, he was concerned about the fact that a large majority of his patients had cavities, crooked teeth and other dental problems, along with skeletal deformities and chronic illness, and he postulated a link with mental illness, mental retardation and juvenile and adult criminal behavior, which were becoming more and more common in urban society.

Dr. Price began a decade-long study, which took him to many isolated parts of the globe, in order to answer two questions. He first wanted to know whether healthy populations existed—populations with excellent dental health, and, by inference, excellent overall health. Secondly, he wanted to know what the diets of healthy people were like. What kinds of foods did they eat? He found fourteen isolated groups worldwide who had freedom from tooth decay, excellent dental structure (wide jaws and straight teeth) and good overall health. Their diets had not changed for centuries. He found that these populations—from the isolated Swiss, Irish and North American Indians to Eskimos, Peruvian Indians, Australian Aborigines and Africans—experienced vibrant health generation to generation. They were free of chronic disease, dental decay and crowding, skeletal deformities, mental illness and retardation. They also produced healthy children with ease. Today, it would be nearly impossible to carry out this kind of study, as nearly every country in the world has been exposed to refined and industrialized food.

Dr. Price found that although the diets of these populations differed in details, they contained important characteristics in common. Almost without exception, the groups he studied consumed generous amounts of seafood or other animal proteins and fats in the form of organ meats and raw dairy products. They emphasized fats as indispensable to good health, and they ate fats, meats, legumes, nuts, seeds, vegetables, fruits and whole grains in their whole and unrefined state.

He had numerous opportunities to observe the consequences when people began to consume foods of the industrial revolution—refined grains, canned foods, pasteurized milk and sugar. These people experienced extensive tooth decay, infectious disease and degenerative illness and, in the next generation, crooked teeth, narrowed faces and other deformities of bone structure. He also found that when these same people returned to their native diets they recovered from their serious illnesses. Good bone structure resulting in straight teeth returned in the next generation.

In applying these nutritional principles to his patients, Price was able to help them reverse tooth decay and chronic illness. Furthermore, he found that if a prospective set of parents ate a diet based on these principles before conceiving, and the mother continued the diet during pregnancy, they would have healthy children who were free of any skeletal deformities including dental crowding, even though they themselves had this very problem. Good nutrition practice, therefore, can correct physical deformities considered genetic.

As early as the 1930s, Dr. Price clearly understood the fact that continued use of refined and industrialized foods would result in a dramatic increase in chronic disease, skeletal deformities, mental problems and even infertility. Need I say that his insight was profound? And if we compare the food quality in 1930 to that of today, with our meats, poultry, eggs, and dairy produced by the industrial farming system, we can see a continued decline in food quality with exactly the results he predicted.

Price's studies of healthy populations determined several basic nutritional elements necessary for optimal health. Regardless of dietary differences, these important factors were present in all the groups he studied.

The prevailing element in the diets of healthy populations was the presence of what he called "fat-soluble activators," vitamins A and D, abundantly present in raw butterfat produced by cows feeding on rapidly growing grass, as well as in seafood, fish-liver oils, fish eggs, egg yolks from chickens on pasture, organ meats from animals eating a species-appropriate diet, blubber of sea animals and insects. Traditional cultures valued these as sacred foods.

Fat-soluble activators are critical to health because they are catalysts for the absorption of vitamins, minerals and protein. In other words, you cannot make use of the building blocks in your food (minerals, vitamins and amino acids) without the "fat-soluble activators" carried uniquely in these foods. Dr. Price found that the nutrient content of native diets consisted of *ten* times more of these fat-soluble vitamins than the American diet in the 1930s—the difference would be even greater today as we have abandoned animal fats and organ meats as unhealthy. Without these important fat-soluble vitamins, the body is unable to obtain adequate nutrients from food, no matter how otherwise nutritious the diet.

Dr. Price also discovered the extraordinary healing properties in the combination of high-vitamin cod liver oil given with high-vitamin butter oil, which together are very high in the fat-soluble activators, vitamins A and D. He successfully used this therapy to increase the nutrient absorption of foods and reverse many disease conditions.

Adequate presence of vitamins A and D assures fertility, healthy growth in children, healthy bones, proper development of the brain and nervous system, a healthy gastro-intestinal tract, beautiful bone structure, wide palate, and flawless, uncrowded teeth. These fat-soluble nutrients also help heal the gut and prevent and correct degenerative conditions such as inflammatory processes, digestion problems and arthritis.

Thus, by focusing on obtaining ample amounts of vitamins A and D, as an adjunct to establishing a healthy intestinal ecosystem and a healthy diet, many of the common degenerative and inflammatory conditions that musicians, athletes, dancers and others experience may be alleviated as the body is able to garner more nutrients from foods. This was my experience. Through the nutritional principles of Dr. Price, I went from a condition of severe inflammation, embouchure shaking, malabsorption and malnutrition to one characterized by freedom from pain and inflammation, stability in my embouchure muscles, excellent stamina and a feeling of strength.

I must add though, that I had to be very disciplined. Dr. Jordan Rubin compares the people who overcome chronic illness to the people who make it to the Olympics. The process of healing with a nutritional approach takes time, patience, persistence and knowledge. At times, I felt as though I would not survive my illness—as though I were hanging from a skyscraper by one arm—but, eventually, I did more than recover; I became exceptionally healthy. I, like you, have the desire to enjoy my life and my career for many years to come. This goal was well worth the price of the required discipline.

Dr. Price's work provides a timeless guide to human health. Through his inspiring studies, we can correct our nutritional deficits, move towards a state of vibrant well-being and secure these principles for generations to come.

# 4

# *FOODS TO AVOID*

C ertain foods are highly problematic for the proper functioning of the digestive system. An impaired digestive system may predispose you to degenerative conditions, including recurring inflammatory symptoms, and take significant energy away from the repair and maintenance of the body. For musicians, athletes and dancers, these foods use up energy needed for repair and maintenance of the critical muscles and tendons necessary for injury-free performance. Untreated digestive disorders may eventually lead to serious illness.

## GLUTEN-CONTAINING GRAINS

Today's gluten-containing grains (wheat, barley and rye) can present serious health issues for all of us. Historically, many degenerative disease-free cultures ate no grains whatsoever, and those that did eat grains soaked, sprouted or fermented them before preparing them into breads, porridges and beverages. Through this process, the difficult-to-digest gluten protein and mineral-blocking components in grains are broken down. The result is enhanced digestibility and nutritional value. However, today's massive consumption of refined, quickly prepared and unfermented high-gluten grains puts an incredible strain on our digestive systems. A compromised digestive system can lead to many degenerative health conditions. For instance, musicians and athletes with digestive issues may experience weakness, instability and a predisposition to inflammatory conditions of the muscles, ligaments and tendons as the body withholds repair energy from these less important physiological functions.

Many health practitioners have found that when improperly prepared or refined grains are consumed, they are only partially digested, causing some of the unabsorbed carbohydrates to remain in the small intestines. When this regularly occurs, harmful bacteria, can colonize the intestinal tract and upset the balance of intestinal flora. As a result, *Candida albicans*, a yeast fungus which normally exists in balance with the other microorganisms in the intestines, over-multiplies and changes from a beneficial yeast to a harmful fungus. These harmful microbes consume the undigested carbohydrates, leading to bacterial and fungal fermentation. This can result in intestinal damage such as bowel problems and intestinal wall permeability—called "leaky gut syndrome"—where proteins and other food components can leak through the intestinal lining into the bloodstream and cause a susceptibility to common health problems such as food allergies (even to healthy foods), irritable bowel syndrome, chronic fatigue, skin problems, intestinal bloating and cramping. The body reacts to these leaked substances as "foreign invaders" and produces antibodies against them. This creates a cascade of biochemical events that ultimately increase the levels of inflammatory prostaglandins in your tissues, leading to an increase in pain. The amazing fact is that pain is not confined to the intestines. Because the inflammatory chemicals circulate throughout the body, a person can develop muscle, joint, tendon and even headache pain.

Dr. Turner suggests a simple laboratory test to determine whether you have a leaky gut. Two sugars, one small and one large, are ingested on an empty stomach. A urine sample is collected over the course of 24 hours and then tested for the presence of the two sugars. If there are more of the larger sugars present in the urine, then these sugars were absorbed before being completely broken down, and a leaky gut is present.

The resulting gas and acid from ongoing fermentation in the gut also make digestion of carbohydrates more difficult as the intestines produce excess mucus to fight against these microbial toxins, acids and unabsorbed carbohydrates. This mucus interferes with the digestive enzymes on the intestinal wall, further complicating carbohydrate absorption, ultimately resulting in malnourishment.

Another problem with the consumption of refined grains is that they cause a surge in blood sugar, leading to disruption of critical hormonal balances. Of particular importance to musicians and others engaged in repetitive-motion activity are the hormones for the growth and repair of body tissues. When these hormone balances are upset, the body's ability to maintain and repair itself can be drastically impaired. Furthermore, an increase of insulin occurs with refined carbohydrate consumption, which causes the production of pro-inflammatory prostaglandins (hormone-like substances).

Although the undigestible fiber in grains is thought to promote regularity, it can have negative effects as well. The fiber can cause damage to the mucosal lining of the intestinal wall and also bind with nutrients, making them unavailable.

Finally, refined and improperly prepared grains are quite low in nutritional density, and therefore not good choices for the nutritional requirements necessary for maintaining optimal health.

Proper preparation of grains includes soaking them overnight in acidulated water (water with yogurt, kefir, lemon or vinegar added) or sprouting them. However, when you have grain intolerance and damage to the intestinal mucosal lining, even properly prepared grains will be extremely problematic.

# Performance without Pain

EARLY SIGNS OF GRAIN INTOLERANCE

In the introduction of this book I described the many inflammatory and physical problems I had to overcome in order to keep playing my instrument. My intolerance to gluten-containing grains was the main cause of these serious symptoms. You will want to be on the lookout for the various symptoms I suffered—some merely embarrassing and some downright debilitating—that are possible with undiagnosed celiac disease.

FLATULENCE

When I was born, I had a severe case of colic, even though my mother nursed me in order to provide the best possible nutrition. This was in 1957, when doctors did not know a lot about the causes of this problem. In fact, they tried to blame the mother's inexperience with infants as a primary cause. With colic, my belly would blow up with intestinal gas, and I could not sleep. My mother said I cried in agony almost constantly for three whole months. The doctor said I would eventually outgrow the problem. However, I was so uncomfortable, my mother thought she would try eliminating things from her diet that might be causing a reaction to her breast milk. Nothing seemed to work. In fact, she eliminated everything *except wheat* from her diet. This actually caused my stools to turn green and be coated with a lot of mucus! The doctor suggested that this was caused by my mother eating too many carbohydrates.

After three months of misery, my mother decided to stop nursing, as she felt something in her milk was making me sick. What actually had occurred was a sensitization to gluten from my mother's consumption of refined wheat products, literally from the time I was born. The severe flatulence I experienced is one of the common signs of gluten sensitivity.

Next, I was put on a common formula called Similac and began eating a combination of rice cereal and Pablum, a wheat cereal. At that time "allergies to wheat" seemed as ridiculous as "allergies to water;" few people were considering this issue. Thus, I was exposed to wheat at a very early age. Untreated gluten sensitivity causes intestinal damage. I therefore was developing problems with nutrient absorption from the time I was an infant.

Until I regained my digestive health at age 47, I could not remember a time when I did not experience embarrassing flatulence daily, a sure sign of impaired digestion and overgrowth of harmful bacteria in the intestinal tract. It is also a sign of poor nutrient assimilation, leading to malabsorption and malnourishment. The lesson to keep in mind: this symptom should not be ignored! Early detection and correction of the causes of digestive issues may prevent a much more serious condition from developing later on.

CARBOHYDRATE ADDICTION

Craving for grains is a sign of grain sensitivity and celiac disease. There are certain protein fragments, or peptides, found in gluten that act like the narcotic morphine. They are inactive within the gluten protein but can be released after contact with secretions of the pancreas and stomach. If the grain has not been properly prepared to break down the gluten protein, as in the process of soaking or fermenting, or if it is in a refined form, these protein fragments are highly resistant to enzyme digestion in the intestines. There is much evidence indicating that these morphine-like peptides may be responsible for the many health problems associated with gluten. Some research suggests that these "exorphines," or morphine-like proteins, give a feeling of physical and sensual comfort, which leads to overconsumption. Because exorphines are biochemically similar to heroin, cocaine and morphine, untreated celiac patients experience powerful cravings leading to food addictions.

I remember having addict-like cravings for wheat. Throughout my childhood I remember seeking out gluten foods to satisfy hunger. When I was in undergraduate school, I worked in a whole-wheat doughnut shop for a year and regularly binged on copious amounts of these delicious pastries, thinking that they were "healthy" because they were made from whole wheat. In the 1980s, the USDA recommended breads, cereals and pasta, as "most important" in the Food Pyramid, so naturally I concluded that eating a lot of wheat, especially whole-wheat products, was very nutritious. I ate lots of pasta and fell in love with bagels, often eating 2-3 bagels every day. A pan of brownies was absolutely irresistible!

WEIGHT GAIN

A by-product of my addiction to gluten grains was a constant battle with my weight. I gained weight very easily. In my freshman year of both high school and college, I gained many pounds. For instance, in my first year of undergraduate music school, when I worked at the whole-wheat doughnut shop, I went from 125 pounds to 168 pounds. I am five-feet four-inches tall, so that was quite a jump. Unfortunately, because I gained weight so easily, after my freshman year in college, I was determined never to be fat again, so I often would limit my intake of meats and fat, and just eat salads, vegetables and bread with a small amount of protein. According to the recommendations of the Food Pyramid, a more "vegetarian" diet was perfectly healthy. I was able to maintain my weight at about 120 pounds for many years, but only through strictly limiting my food intake and getting regular exercise. I stayed thin by eliminating some of the most densely nutritious foods, which may well have added to my malnourishment problems.

Today we know more about high-carbohydrate diets and fat accumulation. High-carbohydrate foods trigger a strong insulin response, which leads to the accumulation of body fat. Significantly, these foods tend to be low in fiber, protein, important fatty acids, and vitamins and minerals that either buffer the absorption of carbohydrates or aid in their metabolism.

DEPRESSION

Some researchers believe that depression is one of the most common symptoms of grain sensitivities. I struggled with depression during my childhood and early adulthood, while regularly eating foods containing gluten. My solace was to practice the clarinet, which helped soothe my soul. However, during the time when I went through a lot of auditions, I often thought of ending my life, as the process made me feel so insignificant. Luckily my family, friends and spirituality held me together.

EATING DISORDERS

Another early symptom of gluten sensitivity was an eating disorder. Throughout my childhood, teenage years and adulthood, I often experienced huge mood swings. These were especially prevalent during the years I was in post graduate school and the three subsequent years spent playing in the Chicago Civic Orchestra.

When I was working on my Doctorate in Clarinet Performance at Indiana University and beginning to take auditions, I had wonderful playing opportunities as Principal Clarinet in the top orchestra. I was practicing four to six hours a day in addition to rehearsals and classes. As excited as I was about the wonderful music I was performing, I had a very dark and private side of my life. I began to develop bulimia. When I was depressed, I would binge on ice cream and sweets. But I did not want to gain weight, so I would purge this food.

This secret habit went on for about two years until I began talking about it with my family and a fellow clarinetist who played with me in the Chicago Civic Orchestra. She, too, was bulimic and needed support to help her through this devastating habit. Through talking about our problems, we learned to find other ways to deal with the frustrations of our pursuit. When we felt the surge of stress, rather than turning to unhealthy foods, we discussed our issues and strictly limited foods that contained sugar. This helped thwart our self-destructive patterns. We both eventually were able to overcome this serious life-threatening eating disorder.

I learned from my studies that eating disorders are common symptoms of gluten allergy. Today's increased incidence of eating disorders may be related to the increased incidence of grain sensitivities.

CAVITIES

When I was in high school, I suddenly got cavities inside every one of my molars. Cavities are a sign of poor health. With undiagnosed grain sensitivities, imbalanced intestinal bacterial flora and intestinal damage developing, my body was not obtaining adequate nutrients from the foods that I was eating. My diet also did not have the necessary high-quality proteins, vitamins A and D, nutrient density and saturated fats to support my growth. As Dr. Price found in all the cultures that he studied, when people turned to eating refined and denatured foods, their health deteriorated and they developed rampant tooth decay. When the body has insufficient calcium and phosphorus stores, which result from an inadequate diet, it begins to pull minerals away from the teeth and bones to fulfill physiological requirements. Poor digestion and inadequate diet create the scene for tooth decay—a signal not to be ignored!

MUSCLE ACHES AND BONE PAINS

From the time I was a child, I frequently felt aches in muscles and bones, sometimes quite severe, especially in my legs and back. From my research, I learned that this symptom is common to grain intolerance as well. It stems from inadequate levels of vitamins, minerals—especially calcium—and nutrients, which can be a consequence of malabsorption caused by intestinal damage.

SKIN PROBLEMS

Lastly, I experienced frequent skin rashes and dry skin problems on my scalp and body. My skin was often irritated, flaky and itchy. Constant applications of lotion offered only temporary relief. These irritations were yet additional symptoms of poor digestion and malnourishment caused by food allergy.

A HEALTHY APPROACH TO GRAIN CONSUMPTION

Because of the many problems associated with gluten-containing grains, we recommend completely removing them from your diet

# 4. Foods to Avoid

for a period of time, even if you think you have no trouble digesting them. Excellent health starts with digestion and a healthy intestinal ecosystem; both are necessary for the assimilation of nutrients. To begin this process, it is essential to replace grains with foods that are higher in nutrients and that do not irritate the digestive tract. This will also give the digestive system the nourishment it needs to heal.

After a period of avoidance, you will be able to assess your health more accurately. If you find that you feel much better you probably have undiagnosed gluten intolerance and will want to continue the practice of a gluten-free diet indefinitely. The earlier you detect this problem, the better.

Once your digestion has improved, you may try including small amounts of properly prepared whole grains to your diet. There are several brands of sourdough bread available that are made from sprouted grains, but be careful. Sprouting and sour leavening may make the grains more digestible but often manufacturers add gluten before baking, so read labels! (See Sources for recommended breads.) Grains and flours prepared at home should be soaked in warm acidulated water (water with yogurt, kefir, buttermilk, whey, lemon juice or vinegar added) for at least seven hours before cooking or baking (see recipes in Chapter 9.) This process allows enzymes, lactobacilli and other helpful organisms to break down the difficult-to-digest gluten proteins and also neutralize enzyme inhibitors and phytic acid, a substance in grains that blocks mineral absorption.

However, be very observant: if you feel *any* symptoms of digestive difficulty after trying properly prepared grains, you should consider leaving them out of your diet longer, perhaps indefinitely. You may want to have a test done for gluten sensitivity—there are new blood tests that are very accurate and can diagnose both gluten sensitivity and celiac disease.

If you are grain intolerant, you may find a cautious use of rice crackers and gluten-free breads helpful. However, I found the total elimination of grains, in favor of more nutritious foods, offered the greatest health benefits.

SUGAR AND HIGH FRUCTOSE CORN SYRUP

Avoiding sugar and high fructose corn syrup is crucial to preventing injury and improving your health. These refined carbohydrates cause the same bacterial and hormonal imbalances as refined grains and may ultimately impair the body's ability to repair and maintain tissues. They alter immune function and lead to a predisposition to inflammation. They also disturb blood sugar levels, causing a sharp rise in blood sugar followed by a plummet. When these swings in blood sugar levels occur regularly, they can negatively affect virtually every function of the body. Since the refinement of grains and carbohydrates strips them of their nutrients, digestion of these refined carbohydrates calls on the body's own reserves of vitamins, minerals and enzymes for proper metabolism. The consumption of refined sweeteners can therefore seriously affect the muscle and tendon function of musicians, athletes and dancers, who require significant metabolic energy for their use, repair and maintenance—energy that may not be available when there are physiological imbalances.

Refined sweeteners were unknown in the human diet before 1600 and were rarely used in great quantities before the twentieth century. For example, in 1821, the average American consumed 10 pounds of sugar per year; today it is 170 pounds per person—or over one-fourth of the caloric intake!

Not only can sugar be a factor in the predisposition to inflammation, it has been linked to kidney disease, liver disease, shortened life span, cancer, overgrowth of *Candida albicans*, bone loss, tooth decay, atherosclerosis and coronary heart disease.

High fructose corn syrup, another widely used sweetener, especially in soft drinks, produces the same problems as does refined sugar, plus it has been shown to interfere with the formation of collagen. Collagen is an important component of supple skin, flexible tendons and connective tissue.

A very limited use of natural sweeteners, such as raw honey, date sugar, maple syrup and dehydrated cane juice as part of whole foods desserts, is usually not problematic. However, if you are experiencing any problems with digestion, inflammation or other degenerative conditions, eliminating all forms of sugar, even natural sugar, will support your recovery.

TOO MUCH FIBER FROM GRAINS AND FIBER SUPPLEMENTS

As we have discussed, the fiber in improperly prepared grains can cause intestinal damage. Eating a high-fiber diet as recommended can initiate digestive disorders and malnourishment. Diets high in hard-to-digest grains are low in nutrient density and can foster nutrient deficiencies.

Conventional nutritionists tell us that a high-fiber diet is good for digestive health, when in fact, because our modern diets lack the basic elements for good digestion, fiber from too many whole grains and especially fiber supplements may actually cause digestive problems. During digestion, fiber can expand the digestive tract beyond its normal size. Eventually intestinal damage and bowel problems can develop, including hernias, hemorrhoidal disease, constipation, malnourishment, irritable bowel syndrome and Crohn's disease. The continual irritation of this fiber expansion may also compromise the delicate protective intestinal mucosal lining and become a factor in the development of leaky-gut syndrome. Additionally, instead of aiding the digestive process, excess fiber slows it down and causes fermentation in the gut, contributing to bacterial flora imbalances in the intestinal tract. These bacterial imbalances make it difficult for your body to break food down and absorb nutrients.

Many people seek fiber supplements to correct constipation. However, these supplements do not correct the intrinsic problem of gut damage and basic deficiencies. Often these supplements just make the problem worse.

Our ancestors could handle a certain amount of fiber because they had healthy digestive tracts and because they prepared high-fiber food properly. The modern combination of lowfat, nutrient-deficient diets with lots of high-fiber food has led to widespread suffering from digestive disorders.

FRUIT JUICES AND HIGH-SUGAR FRUITS

Americans love fruit and fruit juices. Health-conscious people think fruit and juices for breakfast, snacks and dessert are ideal. Fruit, however, played a very small role in the diets of our ancestors. Fruits were traditionally eaten only in season and fruit juice was virtually unknown. Today pasteurized fruit juice, void of enzymes, high in sugar and high in pesticides, is a daily dietary component for many people. Fruit juices and high-sugar fruits such as oranges, bananas and grapes can often aggravate or create intestinal disorders as they upset the healthy bacterial intestinal flora, leading to flatulence and indigestion. The nutrients and antioxidants found in fruit may be equally supplied by other foods, such as vegetables and animal fats like butter.

Fresh, low-sugar, whole fruit, such as berries, are fine in moderation especially when consumed with a healthy fat such as cream or whole coconut milk. High-pectin fruits such as apples, pears, apricots and peaches can cause intestinal problems in sensitive people and are best eaten cooked (sautéed or stewed). Once you are accustomed to a native diet, the desire for fruit will likely fade, as other foods will satisfy your nutrient requirements. Then you will be satisfied with small amounts of fruit in season.

SUGAR SUBSTITUTES

Sugar substitutes, which have become extremely popular, particularly in soft drinks, have many dangers that can affect your health. The most widely used artificial sweetener is aspartame—sold as Equal or Nutra-Sweet—which is a neurotoxic substance that has been linked with numerous serious health problems such as dizziness, visual impairment, severe muscle aches, numbing of the extremities, pancreatitis, high blood pressure, retinal hemorrhaging, seizures and depression. And these artificial sweeteners won't even reduce the craving for sweets or aid in weight loss. In fact, in animal studies, aspartame caused obesity.

The newest sweetener on the market is called sucralose or Splenda.

# 4. Foods to Avoid

Although sucralose has not been thoroughly researched, recent studies indicate that it may enlarge the kidneys and liver and cause the thymus to shrink. With years or decades of use, it may contribute to serious chronic immunological or neurological disorders.

Because of the problems associated with sugar substitutes, we recommend eliminating them from your diet.

COMMERCIAL DAIRY PRODUCTS

Modern commercial dairy foods are frequently problematic. For 30,000 years, milk—a highly nutrient-dense food—was consumed in its natural raw state, providing health benefits for countless cultures worldwide. This healthy milk came from cows on pasture. However, most of today's cows are kept in confinement systems and fed a grain-based diet with many unhealthy additives. The milk is pasteurized, which destroys the enzymes and natural healthy bacteria that help to make the milk proteins easily digestible and alters the amino acids lysine and tyrosine, making the whole complex of protein less available. Pasteurization also greatly diminishes vitamin C and the other water-soluble vitamins, and reduces the availability of macro and trace minerals. In addition, homogenization transforms the fats in milk, making them more susceptible to rancidity. For these reasons, commercial milk puts undue strain on the digestive system, nullifying its original attributes.

VEGETABLE OILS

Avoiding vegetable oils (in both liquid and partially hydrogenated forms) and replacing them with traditional fats will help you move past inflammatory tendencies. Vegetable oils have been shown to contribute to digestion problems and inflammation.

Since 1950, an entire new class of vegetable fats began to replace the traditional saturated fats that had nourished people for thousands of years. Groups with backing from the vegetable oil industry, such as the American Heart Association and research departments at major universities, created a theory that high cholesterol causes heart disease and promoted a false notion that vegetable oils and lowfat diets are healthier. These unfortunate fallacies have had an extremely negative effect on our food supply. "Fat-free" foods, "lowfat" foods, processed foods made with partially hydrogenated vegetable oils, margarine, spreads and foods containing processed polyunsaturated vegetable oils, replaced butter, full-fat dairy foods and traditional fats such as lard, tallow and coconut oil. As a result, several generations of consumers have been missing very critical nutritional elements that were previously provided by traditional fats.

Vegetable oils such as corn, safflower, peanut, soy and cottonseed oils contain mostly omega-6 fatty acids. In traditional diets there was a close ratio between the omega-6 fatty acids and the omega-3 fatty acids (no more than 4:1 and often as close as 1:1). Today, omega-6 fatty acids dominate omega-3 fatty acids by ratios estimated between 20:1 and 30:1! Research indicates that too much omega-6 in our diet causes an imbalance in the production of important hormones called prostaglandins, which can lead to a propensity toward inflammation as well as other serious health problems. Not only have we been encouraged to use these high-omega-6 oils, but we have also added to the imbalance by eating poultry, eggs and fish from animals raised in confinement on a grain-based diet instead of their traditional pasture-based diet. When fish and chicken are raised in confinement, they end up with mostly omega-6 fatty acids in the tissues and eggs.

Another reason polyunsaturates cause so many health problems is because they become rancid or oxidized when subjected to heat and oxygen during processing. Rancid oils contain free radicals, which are extremely reactive chemically and can damage cells and accelerate the aging process.

In addition, diets high in fats from vegetable sources lack adequate amounts of saturated fat necessary for the body to function properly. Saturated fats play a vital role in digestion and assimilation of nutrients, in calcium metabolism, in the integrity of cell walls throughout the body including the intestinal wall—integrity necessary to prevent "leaky gut syndrome"—in muscle and tendon repair and maintenance, in brain function, in lung function, in cell function, in hormone regulation and in the protection against harmful microorganisms in the digestive tract. Our bodies simply cannot function properly without adequate amounts of traditional saturated fats!

After World War II, hydrogenated vegetable oils replaced coconut and animal fats in processed foods, marketed as "healthy" alternatives to saturated fats. These *trans* fats mimic the characteristics of saturated animal fats in their cooking properties, but most of these man-made *trans* fats are toxins to the body. Unfortunately, your digestive system does not recognize them as such, so they are readily incorporated into the cell membranes where they can cause problems with cell metabolism leading to inflammation and pain.

To successfully avoid polyunsaturated and hydrogenated vegetable oils, you must read labels. You will find that most of the foods at the grocery store and fast food restaurants contain these types of oils.

TOO MANY RAW VEGETABLES

Although raw vegetables are considered healthful by today's standards, just as with grains and fiber supplements, they may pose problems for those whose digestion is impaired in any way. Eating too many raw vegetables can irritate the digestive track, and nutrients from raw vegetables are very difficult to assimilate when digestion has been compromised.

Our ancestors ate comparatively few raw vegetables because for most cultures, they were available only in the summer season. During harvest, many vegetables were preserved through lacto-fermentation or cooked in bone-broth soups.

I am now convinced that my habit of eating fresh raw vegetables in the form of at least one large raw salad a day plus raw snacks played a large part in my illness.

One of my first symptoms of digestive illness was acid-reflux disease—often a sign of a hiatal hernia, where part of the stomach is pushed up through the diaphragm into the esophagus. This can be caused by an injury, but often it develops as a result of constant intestinal gas from fermentation in the gut, which puts undue pressure on the entire digestive system. Eventually the diaphragm weakens, and the stomach pushes up towards the esophagus, allowing stomach acid to easily escape into the esophagus and producing an uncomfortable feeling of pressure in the throat as well. Left untreated, a person with chronic heartburn can develop esophageal problems and swallowing difficulties.

Cutting out wheat controlled my first symptoms of acid reflux. However, after I had recovered for several years through a nutrient-dense diet, which, as previously mentioned, was low in fiber, I started adding raw vegetables back into my diet, thinking I could now consume them. After two months, I was again experiencing acid-reflux— a sign that my hiatal hernia was causing symptoms. I came to the conclusion that raw vegetables were the culprit. When I removed them, these symptoms disappeared immediately. *Oh, if I only had four stomachs like a cow, I could munch on raw salad without a care!* But, I'd rather enjoy good health. It is difficult to recover from digestive problems if you continue to consume raw vegetables.

If you're worried about getting enough nutrients in your diet without raw vegetables, remember that animal foods from pastured animals contain concentrated nutrients because the animals spend their whole lives chowing down literally bushels of fresh green grass and other plant matter. The result is meat and fat containing all the vitamins and minerals found in fresh produce, not only in more concentrated form, but also one that is easier to digest.

Don't worry—you can still enjoy vegetables. Just make sure they are lacto-fermented, used in bone broth soups or steamed and served with butter. Cooking breaks down indigestible fiber—that's one reason why human beings cook their food.

## 4. Foods to Avoid

RAW VEGETABLE JUICES

Just as with fruit juices, overconsumption of vegetable juices can cause the upset of the acid-alkaline balance of the body, making it too alkaline. This can promote the growth of harmful bacteria in the gut. Plus, these juices provide very little nourishment.

TOO MUCH WATER

We often hear that we must faithfully drink eight glasses of water a day, or we will not be hydrated. But what you may not realize is that this modern practice can cause problems such as constipation, mineral depletion and imbalances, which can contribute to digestive disorders, kidney disease, degenerative bone disease, muscular disorders and even cardiac arrest from electrical dysfunction. Biochemistry textbooks tell us that when we drink a large quantity of water, this upsets the body's homeostasis; the body reacts by getting rid of the water as quickly as it can.

Interestingly, on the cellular level, your body makes its own water during the metabolism of the food—especially fat—you eat. Because modern diets tend to be low in fats, people often experience a sense of thirst. And because we consume less fat and eat no traditional fermented foods, many people tend to have problems with constipation. Drinking more water does not prevent this problem, as we've been told; water is transported through the kidneys and does not hydrate the bowels. To ensure healthy elimination, we need fats, the proper mineral balance and plentiful healthy intestinal bacteria. Thus, if we drink excess amounts of water and do not eat foods that aid in good digestion, we may upset our mineral balances and actually become constipated.

Historically, people did not drink large quantities of water because a clean water source was not guaranteed. Instead, they stayed hydrated because their diets included ample traditional fats and they consumed dairy, fermented beverages and bone broth soups, all of which have incredible nutrient qualities and are not flushed through the body as plain water.

As a guide, limit total water intake—including water in foods—to 8 cups a day. If you increase your traditional fat intake and choose high-quality dairy, fermented beverages and bone-broth soups, you will find that your hydration will improve along with your digestion.

FLUORIDATED AND CHLORINATED WATER

Fluoridated and chlorinated water should be avoided, even in small quantities. Fluoride is an enzyme inhibitor that can cause bone loss, bone deformities, cancer and other illnesses. It offers little protection against tooth decay, which is really caused from eating refined foods. Drinking chlorinated water can destroy the body's healthy bacterial flora. Be sure to use only filtered water for cooking and drinking (see Sources).

FOODS AND BEVERAGES MADE FROM
SOY, WHEY, CASEIN AND EGG WHITES

Soy foods and beverages have recently received enormous positive press from the media, many health practitioners and health books. Soy is advertised as a highly nutritious protein, a wonderful alternative to milk and an aid for women to prevent menopause symptoms and bone loss. Unfortunately, the funding for this research has come from the soybean industry—and so should be viewed with great skepticism.

Historically, traditional societies who consumed soybeans did so by fermenting them to produce foods such as *miso, natto* and *tempeh.* This important process is necessary for the body to assimilate the nutrients in the soybean. A long period of fermentation breaks down soy's difficult-to-digest phytates and enzyme inhibitors. Furthermore, Asian societies consumed these foods only in small amounts, and not as a substitute for animal foods.

Commercial soy beverages and protein powders, however, are made from unfermented soy or refined soy protein isolates that are processed at high temperatures, which denature them, making their nutrients and proteins indigestible. They are also high in mineral-blocking phytates, thyroid-depressing phytoestrogens and potent enzyme inhibitors that inhibit digestion and may be a factor in cancer.

Tofu, another popular soy food, contains a high phytate content, making it a poor protein substitute. It is best consumed in small amounts in fish broth as in traditional Japanese cuisine.

Other protein isolates such as whey, casein and egg white are also denatured and over-processed. They are not good substitutes for high-quality traditional proteins in meat, fish, milk products, eggs and organ meats. In fact, diets in which unnatural isolated powdered proteins from soy, eggs or milk are fed to animals or humans cause a negative calcium balance that can lead to osteoporosis.

An excellent, extremely nutritious and delicious substitute for milk is whole coconut milk with dolomite powder added for calcium (see Sources). Coconut products have been traditional foods for healthy cultures for millennia. (See Chapter 5 and recipes in Chapter 9.)

COFFEE AND TEA

For anybody with digestive issues, coffee and other caffeinated beverages are highly problematic, as they inhibit proper digestive and adrenal function. Caffeine is an irritant to the stomach and esophagus. It relaxes the sphincter muscle that allows food to pass from the esophagus to the stomach, thus permitting hydrochloric acid from the stomach to enter the esophagus, causing heartburn. And caffeine can tax the adrenal glands, thus weakening the immune system and making the body more susceptible to illness.

Switching to highly nutritious beverages (see Chapter 5) and herbal teas (without barley malt if you are gluten sensitive) will be an important aspect of your recovery program.

ALCOHOL

Alcohol can hamper progress in healing from a digestive disorder. Alcohol, like coffee, relaxes the esophageal sphincter and can cause heartburn. It also depletes the body of nutrients. It is best to avoid alcohol completely during your recovery for at least eight to twelve months, and strictly limit alcohol intake to small amounts of wine or unpasteurized beer (not for those with grain intolerance) once you are much better.

ADDITIVES—ESPECIALLY MSG

There are multitudes of additives that have found their way into our food supply: preservatives, artificial and natural flavorings, texture enhancers and colorings. We encourage you to avoid them, as combinations of these substances can be toxic.

MSG or hydrolyzed protein is particularly problematic. MSG is ubiquitous in processed foods and not always clearly labeled. It is listed as "hydrolyzed protein" in items such as soy-based products, dehydrated soups and meat-broth substitutes. MSG is always found in calcium caseinate, sodium casienate, textured protein and citric acid; soy foods, nutritional yeasts, protein powders, malt flavorings and amino acids. Various mixes labeled "flavorings," "natural flavors" or "seasonings" usually contain MSG. Even reduced-fat milk contains this neurotoxin! "Just add water" soups, often a staple for those who eat out of vending machines, are just loaded with MSG, and it is often formed during processing even if it is not deliberately added.

MSG is an unnatural chemical compound that causes neurological reactions in many people and can be a contributing factor in pain.

As a rule of thumb, it is best to prepare your foods at home with natural spices. However, if on occasion you purchase packaged foods, avoid those containing an ingredient list that only a chemist can understand!

MICROWAVED FOODS

The microwave oven has become the fast-paced person's answer to home cooked meals in a "jiffy"! Unfortunately, the effects of microwaves on nutrients in foods were not investigated before these ovens hit the popular market. Research indicates that fats and proteins in microwaved foods are more difficult to assimilate, and vitamin content and availability may be altered. Muscle-testing techniques suggest that microwaved foods contribute to fatigue. Much fast food and restaurant food is microwaved. Even if you are eating in a gourmet restaurant, ask before you order! We recommend avoiding microwaved food at all costs.

EATING TOO QUICKLY

In our fast-paced schedules, we can often forget that the food we are eating is required to support our much-needed energy. Good digestion begins in the mouth with saliva thoroughly mixing with our food. When we gulp our food, it causes inordinate stress on a healthy digestive process. Our digestive system then has to break down and assimilate large pieces of underchewed food. Over time, this habit can degrade proper digestive function, cause depletion of metabolic enzymes that are intended for the repair and maintenance of the body, and greatly reduce available nutrients from foods. Thoroughly chewing your food will tremendously enhance its nutritive value and help to give you vitality.

# 5
# FOODS THAT HEAL

*A*voiding unhealthy foods is only half of the recovery equation. You will also need to embrace a diet based on nutrient-dense foods. The following foods will help heal your digestive system, enable your body to mend, strengthen your muscles and tendons and provide you with the energy you need for peak performance.

A gentle reminder: nutritional healing takes dedication, persistence and patience. At first it will seem very hard—you have to think about everything that you eat and ask yourself, will this food build my health, or will it take away from my progress? You may not experience noticeable results in one or two months, but if you persevere, you should feel improvement after six months. Your best prospect of recovery will be through following *all* of the details of this program. After some time, your efforts will become routine, and the diet will not seem difficult at all, but simply the natural way to eat. And remember, you can't perform without your body. . . nor can you fulfill your aspirations and enjoy life to its fullest without your health!

RAW AND FERMENTED DAIRY

Clean, whole raw milk from cows raised on pasture will provide you with a source of outstanding nutrition matched by few foods. Most people who have allergies to milk or are lactose intolerant usually do very well on this type of milk because it contains all the natural enzymes that help digest the proteins and sugars in milk. Goat's milk is also a highly nutritional option and, for some people, is tolerated better than cow's milk. With the help of the Weston A. Price Foundation, you should be able to locate a source in your area. This milk can be consumed raw or fermented with a yogurt or kefir starter to further enhance its digestibility and promote a healthy intestinal bacterial flora. Real milk—whole, full-fat and unprocessed, from cows eating fertile pasture—provides nutrient density, enzymes and beneficial lactic acid-producing bacteria necessary for building optimal health.

Today's commercial milk and milk products cause problems for most people. This is because the quality of our milk has dramatically changed over the last fifty years with the industrialization of our farming methods. Today's milk undergoes compulsory pasteurization and homogenization—processes that dramatically deform the proteins and fats (making the proteins allergenic) and reduce nutritional quality. Pasteurization destroys the enzymes in milk, making it difficult to digest, and homogenization alters the fat composition, making it highly susceptible to rancidity and oxidation.

This is a tragic situation because for 30,000 years, many cultures worldwide depended on milk as a highly nutritional dietary necessity, and for centuries physicians have used raw milk as a healing agent and builder of health. Hippocrates, Homer, Herodotus and many other observers from cultures throughout the world have proclaimed the curative power of milk. During the nineteenth century, Russian and German physicians successfully prescribed raw milk to cure a multitude of serious illnesses including digestive disorders, asthma, fluid retention, liver diseases, kidney diseases, allergies, and tuberculosis. A

## 5. Foods That Heal

few decades ago, Americans considered milk necessary to health and believed that a safe, plentiful supply was actually vital to our national security. Today, people are finding nutritional answers to healing chronic illness by again obtaining a healthful supply of clean, raw milk from farmers dedicated to traditional methods of dairy farming.

Dr. Weston Price found many cultures that prospered without milk, but they did so by eating nutritionally dense foods that do not appeal to most people in our country—foods such as organ meats, blubber, raw seafood and insects—or foods that take long preparation time, such as bone broths.

The milk-drinking populations he studied drank health-giving raw milk from cows eating a species-appropriate diet—that is, a diet of *grass*! When cows are at pasture, the nutritional quality of milk is superior to that of confined cows. Few consumers realize that the majority of today's cows are raised in confinement and fed primarily a grain-based diet containing many additives, hormones to unnaturally increase milk supply, and other cheap by-products, including recycled human food such as stale candy and gum, potato chips, swill from ethanol production, bakery waste, citrus peel cake laced with neurotoxic pesticides and even nonfoods that are processed into feed, such as chicken manure, chicken feathers, newsprint and cardboard. Obviously such milk is nutritionally inferior and contains many harmful substances that the cow passes through her udder—pesticides, hormones, aflatoxins, *trans* fats and allergenic proteins. Remember how my mother's milk was bad for me because my mother was eating lots of grains.

Most people today are unaware of the benefits of raw milk. We are told that pasteurization is necessary to protect us from disease. If the curative and health-supporting benefits of raw milk are so profound, why do we have compulsory pasteurization? I was astounded to learn about the amazing background to this question in *The Untold Story of Milk*, by Dr. Ron Schmid. He points out that the merits of pasteurization are highly exaggerated. In fact, all outbreaks of salmonella in recent decades—including a 1985 outbreak in Illinois that struck over 14,000 people—were caused by pasteurized milk.

The modern milking machine and stainless steel tank, along with efficient packaging and distribution, make pasteurization totally unnecessary for purposes of sanitation. Raw milk naturally contains numerous components, including lactic acid-producing bacteria, that protect us against pathogens. When pathogens such as *E. coli* are added to raw milk, the good bacteria kill them off. Pasteurization destroys these helpful compounds and organisms, leaving the finished product devoid of any protective mechanisms should harmful bacteria contaminate the supply.

The move to compulsory pasteurization occurred because of severe abuses in dairy farming in the 1800s, resulting in milk that was unfit for human consumption. A consequence of the War of 1812 was a blockade of America's supply of whiskey from the British West Indies. To fill the demand for whiskey, distilleries were built in every major city in America. A large amount of land once used for dairy pasturage was now appropriated for distillery grain production.

The demand for both milk and whiskey was growing rapidly with the tremendous rise in population in major cities. To fulfill the demand for milk, distillery owners created a new type of dairy—an experiment fueled by greed at the expense of the health of countless people. They housed multitudes of cows, tied continuously in close, unsanitary quarters, next to the distilleries and fed them the distillery slop from whiskey production. The cows were then milked in these very unsanitary conditions. This "swill milk system" became incredibly profitable, as it produced more milk at lower cost than any other system.

However, as one can imagine, the swill milk system had many horrible consequences. First, slop is a dreadful food for cows, which leaves them diseased and emaciated. Secondly, the milk is so defective that it lacks the components needed to make butter and cheese. Often chalk was added to make the watery milk look white. The great rise in infant mortality beginning in 1815 corresponded to the era of the distillery dairies. In fact, by 1839, the death rate among children in large cities was almost 50 percent. Diarrhea and tuberculosis were the common fatal illnesses caused by this tainted milk.

In 1842, to remedy this disaster, several doctors founded the Certified Milk Movement. Clean, raw milk, certified from healthy cows, transported by train to the cities, became available. Health officials expressed extreme gratitude for access to this wonderful food. However, the swill dairies continued to operate well into the early 1900s. Thus, for over one hundred years, systems producing wholesome milk and tainted milk existed in parallel. The swill dairies were outlawed at the same time that the officials proposed pasteurization as a solution. The death rate dropped and pasteurization got the credit. In the end, compulsory pasteurization prevailed over certified raw milk, and health officials unanimously condemned Nature's perfect food.

The superior nutrition of real milk—raw, full-fat, and from pastured cows—offers an incredible source of nutrient density. In most cases, people who cannot tolerate commercial milk find raw milk totally agreeable. The effort made to obtain a good source of raw milk will reap high rewards in health benefits.

POSSIBLE PROBLEMS WITH DAIRY OR OTHER HEALING FOODS

Although rare, once in while, a person may not be able to tolerate one of the healing foods or may develop an allergy to one of them after experiencing their health benefits. It is possible to have an allergy, or to develop an allergy to something like raw milk, raw milk kefir or eggs. In fact, allergies to foods happen easily in people today because a large percentage of our population incurs intestinal damage from their diet of modern refined and depleted foods that are high in polyunsaturated oils and low in traditional saturated fats. As we have previously discussed, with this damage, the intestinal wall becomes permeable—called "leaky gut syndrome"—and even when a healing diet is carefully followed, it can take years to heal this condition. With this syndrome, proteins and other components in foods, even healthy foods, can leak through the intestinal wall into the bloodstream. The body may begin to react to these substances as "foreign invaders" and create antibodies against them. When the food is eaten, the body tries to get rid of the substance. Common allergic reactions are diarrhea, upset stomach, fatigue or skin problems.

Most people do extremely well on raw milk products from pastured cows even if they are lactose intolerant, because the enzyme that breaks down lactose—called lactase—is formed by the good bacteria in the milk. Also, the process of fermenting raw milk, as in kefir or yogurt, breaks down much of the lactose, making the milk even easier to digest.

In my case, although drinking raw milk kefir for eight months had helped me to recover from my illness, I developed a sudden intolerance to this healing food. My symptom was severe diarrhea and my ongoing question was, "Where is the bathroom?" Unfortunately, I had a very busy performing schedule at that time. Nothing compares to the experience of having to run to the bathroom five minutes before performing a sonata in front of two hundred people, or having to sit through a grueling six-hour orchestra rehearsal, with countless solos, staring at your watch, waiting for the next break! It took me four frightening weeks to determine the cause of these symptoms. When I discovered that kefir was the culprit, I was astounded and thoroughly disappointed. I couldn't understand what had happened. Once I removed kefir and other dairy products from my diet, I recovered. I was thrilled to feel good again!

Needless to say, this experience baffled me. What would I use as a replacement in my diet that would make up for the dense nutrition of the kefir that I was drinking? I knew that some of the cultures that Dr. Price studied did not drink milk. I also knew that these cultures focused on bone broths, organ meats, or insects! Insects would definitely not become my cuisine, but I enjoyed bone broths and organ meats, especially beef heart and yes—liver! I increased the bone broth soups and organ meats in my diet, and made sure that I ate more raw butter—raw butter, a very important healing food, is usually well tolerated by people who cannot have dairy, because it contains very few milk proteins.

# 5. Foods That Heal

To replace the healing benefit of raw milk kefir, I learned that coconut products such as creamed coconut (see Sources), whole coconut milk beverages and cultured young coconut juice and meat (see recipes in Chapter 9) are extraordinarily nutritious. I also increased my SBO supplementation (see Sources). Goat's milk would have also been an alternative worth trying, but except for raw goat's milk cheese, available in many health food stores, I found it very hard to obtain. These changes were successful strategies in my quest for vibrant health.

I would like to point out that while I suddenly developed an allergy to raw milk dairy, I was again able to consume kefir and other raw dairy products after waiting for 10 months. Sometimes when a food is avoided for a period of time, it may again be tolerated later.

After eating a healing diet for a while, most people experience resolution of bowel problems such as diarrhea or constipation as digestion improves. However, if you have strictly followed the healing diet for a long period, are symptom free, and you suddenly experience diarrhea that lasts longer than a few days, you need to consider the possibility that you may have become allergic to something that you are eating. To calm your system, it is best to go on a diet of chicken soup until your symptoms resolve, and then add foods, one at a time, back into your diet so that you are able to tell whether you are reacting to any of them. (Follow the protocol in *Restoring Your Digestive Health*, by Jordan Rubin and Dr. Joseph Brasco for moving past chronic diarrhea—see Chapter 8.)

## RAW BUTTER AND CREAM

Along with raw milk, raw butter and cream from pastured animals can provide you with the fats that are essential to recovering and maintaining excellent health. Butter and cream from pasture-fed animals are rich in fat-soluble vitamins A, D, K and E. (Remember that Dr. Price found that vitamins A and D were essential to the proper assimilation of the proteins, minerals and other vitamins in the foods we ingest.) Butter and cream will therefore help you heal, as it enhances the nutrition of the foods that you eat. Furthermore, a substance called the Wulzen Factor in raw butter and cream promotes flexibility in muscles and tendons. (The Wulzen Factor is destroyed by pasteurization.) Butter also has the perfect balance of omega-3 and omega-6 fatty acids and therefore helps protect you from inflammation.

Raw butter, which has very few milk proteins, is usually well tolerated, even by those who are lactose intolerant. It is truly a medicinal food, vital for nourishing the central nervous system and digestive tract. Raw butter will aid in healing an inflamed and porous intestinal lining (leaky-gut syndrome), and the fatty acids in raw butter help beneficial microflora adhere to the mucosal lining, where they can colonize.

We suggest freely using butter and cream, especially unheated, in your diet. Butter can be eaten with meat or vegetables, and cream can be added to soups, fruit and vegetables.

For those with extreme intolerance to milk protein, *ghee* or clarified butter (see Sources) is a form of butter in which the milk solids or casein have been removed. Place butter in a small bowl in an oven set at 200 degrees for one-half hour. The butter will melt and foam will rise to the top and form a crust, which should be carefully skimmed or removed by pouring through a strainer lined with cheesecloth.

## ANIMAL PROTEIN, ESPECIALLY ORGAN MEATS

Adequate amounts of animal protein are necessary for healing, as they provide all the essential amino acids necessary for repairing and maintaining organs, nerves, muscles and flesh. You should include carefully selected wild-caught fish, and red meat, organ meats, eggs and poultry from pastured animals.

Our primitive ancestors subsisted on a diet largely composed of meat, fish and fat, augmented with vegetables, fruit, seeds and nuts. In Africa, Dr. Price found that cultures whose diets included significant amounts of animal foods were far healthier than those whose diets were based on grains and legumes. He also found that healthy traditional cultures prized organ meats, such as liver and marrow, which are unusually high in vitamins A and D and other important nutrients. A good practice—one that will build strength and stamina—is to eat liver at least once a week. There are many delicious ways to do this—from liver with bacon to paté.

It is of utmost importance that you choose animal foods from the most healthfully raised sources to ensure the highest nutrient value in the meat and fat you are eating. As we have discussed, foods from animals raised in the confinement factory system will be lacking in many nutrients. These animals are often sick and produce meat, poultry and eggs that are substandard. The local chapters of the Weston A. Price Foundation (see Sources) can help you find farmers dedicated to raising their animals free-range on pasture. The health benefits of carefully chosen animal foods far outweigh their additional cost.

While vegetarianism is promoted as a healthy lifestyle, it will not provide you with adequate protein, fat and vitamins necessary to heal. If a good supply of raw milk, butter and cheese, as well as organic free-range eggs, can be found, it *may* be possible to eat a lacto-ovo vegetarian diet after your symptoms subside, especially if you prepare your grains properly. The vegan diet, however, will not supply you with the nutrition your body will require to move past inflammatory and other degenerative conditions and, in fact, may cause your condition and health to become even worse.

I was particularly interested in a personal vegetarian health story that I read when I was searching for the life-changing book, *Nutrition and Physical Degeneration,* by Dr. Weston Price. I had trouble getting a copy through bookstores or through the internet. I finally attained it through the incredible wellness catalogue of the Radiant Life Company, which provides products and resources for optimal health and sustainable living. I was so impressed with their sense of purpose that I immediately wanted to learn about their founders. Their mission statement reads: "Radiant Life is dedicated to helping people realize the full expression of their genetic potential, as optimal physical development is the foundation for our highest evolution as a species." They preface their mission statement with this critical paragraph:

"Generations of healthy indigenous peoples, living in accordance with natural laws, have proven that humans have the exquisite genetic potential for vibrant, disease-free health and longevity. Tragically, this incredible history is virtually unknown in the Western world—forgotten, lost or ignored. After a century of unprecedented decline in health, we in the West now accept degenerative disease, digestive disorders, osteoporosis, antidepressants and crooked, decaying teeth as normal. As we move into the new millennium, it is time to reclaim the freedom from disease and radiant health that is our birthright."

I was astounded by these statements and knew I had connected with a company founded by dedicated people who were helping to pave an important path for accurate insight into nutritional understanding. Interestingly, the founders of this company, Christapher Cogswell and Marie Bishop, were once strict vegetarians. This is their story:

"Founded in 1996 by Christapher Cogswell and Marie Bishop, Radiant Life was born out of a passion to explore our highest potential for wellness and to share our findings with others. In search of the secrets of radiant health, we were led to believe that a vegetarian diet was the most nutritious and health-promoting diet. We were deeply inspired by the ecological promises of a plant-based diet, and in time adopted what we assumed was also the most morally and spiritually 'evolved' diet of all—veganism. We believed that the perspectives of John Robbins (author of *Diet for a New America)* and others were truly the hallmark of a new paradigm in conscious eating, and that wide-scale conversion to a vegetarian diet offered the greatest hope for our ravaged planet.

"Eventually we took this dietary philosophy a step further and embraced raw, living food, whose preparation techniques maximize life energy and the bioavailability and the assimilation of nutrients. We taught private and public classes in raw living foods preparation and published *The Living Foods Sourcebook.* We enthusiastically shared our philosophy of increasing one's life energy and longevity with what we believed was the most regenerating and life-giving diet available.

# 5. Foods That Heal

"Our dietary experiment took a turn for the worse, however, when Marie began to show signs of pre-diabetes, and had to eat all day long to avoid constant blood sugar crises; Christapher began to lose his thick hair at the age of 27; and both of us were unable to keep weight on. We began to meet others who had similar challenges with long-term vegetarianism and veganism, and who were, like us, being forced to explore other dietary approaches. We began to do more research and through a series of synchronicities, fortunately came across what we now regard as the most important nutritional research of the past century, and perhaps the entire millennium. In 1997 we discovered the work of Dr. Weston Price, a dentist who had chronicled the healthiest isolated, nonindustrialized peoples around the world in the 1930s and 40s. His incredible work, *Nutrition and Physical Degeneration,* marked the beginning of our new journey. Through the Price-Pottenger Nutrition Foundation, Sally Fallon's *Nourishing Traditions,* Ron Schmid's *Traditional Foods Are Your Best Medicine,* as well as a rather provocative book advocating raw meat and raw animal fats for healing, *We Want to Live,* by Aajonus Vonderplanitz, we learned that humans have a long history of omnivorism, and that perfect health has been demonstrated by many traditional peoples through millennia when consuming the nutrient-dense foods our bodies were designed for. For us this information was nothing short of revolutionary, and while it shattered everything we had believed up to this point about what humans need to be healthy, we were forced to listen, out of our urgent desire to be well and to provide the same opportunity to others.

"Given the extraordinary nature of Dr. Price's research, we were stunned that only a handful of people and organizations were even talking about it, let alone knew about it. Our guiding lights were few. *Nourishing Traditions* became our most constant companion, guiding us through our transition to a mixed, omnivorous diet, both raw and cooked, including lacto-fermented foods and, most importantly, animal protein and fat. We noticed significant, positive changes almost immediately. After one month of eating meat and animal fats again, Christapher's hair stopped falling out. We began to slowly regain our normal weight. Marie's severe hypoglycemia improved dramatically. We felt grounded and stronger in ways we had forgotten were possible. After a combined 22 years as vegetarians we knew we were on the right track: the foods our bodies were evolutionarily designed for were offering us the chance to journey back to health.

"As a result of our experiences we reoriented Radiant Life to share with others what we had learned. Central to our newfound understanding was the fact that there is no one diet that is right for everyone. Genetics, ancestry and many other factors that determine one's unique biochemistry, also determine one's equally unique nutritional needs. As Dr. Price discovered, the individual native diets of each indigenous group were as diverse as their cultures and bioregions. Nevertheless, Price did identify common denominators found in every group. One of the most important ones he discovered: high fat-soluble vitamins, found only in animal foods, directly correlated with their superior health and physical development. In fact, Price's greatest disappointment was that he never found any healthy native group existing exclusively on plant foods. There was no historical precedent, nor has there been since, of any healthy populations reproducing generations of healthy children on an exclusively vegetarian diet, devoid of animal foods."

I recommend a high-quality animal protein at every meal, including organ meats twice a week. You should always eat meat with the fat—avoid meats such as the lean cuts and skinless chicken breasts. These foods are critical to your recovery and necessary to maintain a high level of health.

BONE BROTHS

Bone broths, once common fare for traditional cultures worldwide, are made by simmering a variety of different types of bones, meat and vegetables for two to twenty-four hours, with wine or vinegar to help draw out minerals (see recipes in Chapter 9). For millennia, traditional cultures worldwide have prepared this extremely nutritious base for soups, stews and sauces.

# 5. Foods That Heal

Consuming soups made from broths on a daily basis will help you move past a depleted condition. A South American proverb states, "Good broth resurrects the dead!" There are several reasons why this is so. First, bone broths contain easy-to-assimilate nutrients including the minerals of bone (calcium, magnesium and phosphorus), cartilage and marrow; important amino acids; and vitamins from meat, vitamins and minerals from vegetables. Secondly they provide the components of animal cartilage, which will help heal your own cartilage. Finally, bone broths are rich in gelatin, which aids in digestion and helps heal the gut.

Although people believe they are too busy to make food that requires long periods of cooking, broth is one of the most nutritious foods you can consume and well worth the trouble. It is especially beneficial for people who have digestive disorders, as it is extremely easy to digest. The gelatin in broth is hydrophilic, which means that it attracts liquids, including digestive juices, allowing for rapid and effective digestion. Most people are unaware of the benefits of gelatin supplied by broth. It has been used successfully in the treatment of many intestinal disorders, including hyperacidity (a common complaint among those with digestive disorders), colitis and Crohn's disease, and is helpful in chronic disorders such as diabetes, muscular dystrophy and even cancer.

Once a stock is made, you can create a wonderful variety of nourishing soups (see recipes in Chapter 9). Soups made from broth are very convenient to reheat and take along to work in a thermos.

## LACTO-FERMENTED FOODS AND BEVERAGES

Lacto-fermented foods and beverages are important for developing and maintaining a healthy intestinal tract. Some familiar lacto-fermented foods and beverages include yogurt, kefir, traditional sauerkraut, kimchi and pickles. Beverages can also be lacto-fermented. Some of the most healing lacto-fermented beverages are beet kvass and coconut kefir (see recipes in Chapter 9).

Lacto-fermentation is a traditional method of food preservation that involves culturing or fermenting different foods or beverages with lactic-acid-producing bacteria. This culturing results in the enhancement of nutrients, the production of beneficial bacteria necessary to develop and maintain a healthy intestinal flora, and increased digestibility. A universal practice among traditional peoples, lacto-fermentation preserves foods without the benefit of refrigerators, freezers or canning machines, as lactic acid, a byproduct of the fermentation process, inhibits putrefying bacteria. The beneficial lactobacilli organisms in fermented foods and beverages produce a wealth of helpful digestive enzymes, as well as antibiotic and anticarcinogenic substances.

Unfortunately, modern condiments only mimic traditional fermented foods, providing no health benefits. Today's pickles, ketchup, mustard and relish are made with vinegar, which circumvents the healthy traditional fermentation process, and are pasteurized, destroying both the lactobacilli and enzymes.

Preparation of lacto-fermented foods and beverages is quite easy. You can enjoy the beverages throughout the day and small amounts of lacto-fermented foods with meals.

KOMBUCHA

Another beneficial cultured traditional drink, which is gaining wide popularity in the US, is called kombucha. It is an ancient drink from China that is prepared from a culture called *Bacterium iylinum,* often referred to as a "mushroom," which is placed atop a brew of sweetened black tea. The various organisms in the "mushroom" transform the sugars in the tea into beneficial acids. The taste of kombucha varies from slightly acidic to very sour, depending on the length of the fermentation process.

The beneficial acids in kombucha include lactic acid and glucaric acid. These compounds, plus the beneficial organisms in kombucha, support healthy digestion, immune system function and liver detoxification. Glucaric acid helps the body detoxify.

Kombucha tea can be made at home or purchased ready-made (see Sources). If brewing at home, be sure to use glass jars or bowls instead of ceramic, as minerals from a ceramic jar may leach into the kombucha during the fermentation process. Consumption of one 8- to 16-ounce serving daily is recommended. However, if you are on medication or hormone replacement therapy, you should limit yourself to 4 ounces daily. Overconsumption can result in metabolic lactic acidosis and should be avoided.

## EGG, ESPECIALLY EGG YOLKS

Egg yolks are an excellent source of high-quality fat and can be a rich source of fat-soluble activators—vitamins A and D along with some very important fats called EPA and DHA, which are critical to the health of the nervous system and to maintaining mental acuity. Eggs also provide sulfur-containing proteins, critical to many biochemical processes in the body. Of all foods, egg yolk contains the highest levels of choline, a B vitamin crucial to the nervous system. Eggs are also rich in lecithin, a substance that helps the body use cholesterol properly.

Egg quality is, of course, determined by the diet of the chicken. The most nutritious eggs come from pastured chickens, which eat in the sunlight and eat green grass, bugs and worms. These are far superior to the second choice, eggs from organic, "free-range" chickens. Both choices provide a balanced fatty-acid profile of approximately equal amounts of omega-3 and omega-6 necessary to prevent and help heal inflammatory tendencies. However, the pastured eggs will contain more fat-soluble vitamins A and D, as well as DHA, a fatty-acid important for neurological function. Eggs coming from grain-fed chickens can have levels of inflammatory omega-6 as much as 19 times greater than omega-3!

Most people have been accustomed to eating only cooked eggs because of the fear of salmonella, a bacterium that has been the unfortunate consequence of the horrible crowded and unsanitary conditions that industrially raised chickens must endure. Naturally raised chickens produce high-quality eggs free of salmonella. The yolks can be safely eaten raw, keeping all of their enzymes intact (best in smoothies; see recipes in Chapter 9). Raw egg yolks are traditional to many healthy cultures. However, the whites should be eaten cooked, as raw egg whites contain a substance that can interfere with digestion. (You can use the leftover whites to make coconut macaroons.)

We recommend 3-4 egg yolks daily to build health. If you have allergies to egg yolks, increase the amount of organ meats that you eat, and you will be getting the same nutrients.

COCONUT PRODUCTS

Coconut products are a dietary staple in many tropical regions. Although the coconut is relatively low in protein compared to other nuts, it has many other important nutrient attributes. It provides calcium, iron, magnesium, phosphorus, iodine and many trace minerals. Most importantly, coconut oil is rich in medium-chain saturated fats that have potent antiviral, antifungal and anti-microbial properties. Coconut oil is the best dietary source of the 12-carbon fatty acid called lauric acid, which has been shown to inactivate the HIV virus and Herpes simplex virus-1 in *in vitro* studies. Coconut products are very helpful for developing a healthy immune system and intestinal flora, as they are effective against harmful microorganisms such as candida. The fact that coconut oil strengthens the immune system may be why Thailand, where coconut is a very important dietary element, has the lowest cancer rate of fifty countries surveyed by the National Cancer Institute.

Coconut oil, rich in lauric acid and similar anti-microbial fatty acids, can help to kill or disable pathogenic viruses, bacteria and protozoa and is now being used to treat both AIDS and candida. It also helps to control hypoglycemic tendencies as it stabilizes blood sugar. An additional benefit derives from the fact that the fatty acids in coconut oil boost metabolism, improve thyroid function and enhance the immune system.

An easy way to take coconut oil is to melt 1-2 tablespoons of coconut oil in warm water or herbal tea, twice a day. (If you are not used to eating fats, start with just one-fourth teaspoon and build up gradually.)

The best coconut oil is virgin coconut oil from organic coconuts made in the traditional method and available through mail order. You can purchase high-quality organic coconut oil in health food stores. Avoid any coconut oil that has a metallic or burnt taste.

Creamed coconut uses the whole coconut and removes the water. This can be added to smoothies by first dissolving it in warm water, or directly to soups and other recipes to enhance their nutrient value and add a marvelous flavor.

Whole coconut milk (preferably organic) is one of the few canned products we recommend. It can be used as a good substitute for milk (see recipes in Chapter 9 for a healthful and delicious warm Coconut Milk Tonic that can be taken to work in a thermos) and in recipes for soups and other dishes, thereby adding nutritional value. I also enjoy adding whole coconut milk to herbal tea or hot water.

Young coconuts are a highly nutritious food newly available in this country. They are white in color, are soft on the outside and have a large amount of juice (about 1-1/2 cups per young coconut), which is easily accessible by poking a hole through one of the "eyes" found in the outer flesh. This juice can be made into a nutritious fermented beverage (see recipes in Chapter 9) with the same starter powder used to make whole-milk kefir (see Sources). Young coconuts have a tasty meat that is delicious plain or can be fermented into a coconut yogurt and used alone or in smoothies (see recipes in Chapter 9).

NUTS

Nuts are extremely nutritious and provide a perfect snack food if properly prepared. They are rich sources of natural oils, ranging from 60 to 80 percent of their total caloric value, and contain many B complex vitamins and minerals such as calcium, iron, magnesium, phosphorus, potassium and selenium. Traditional peoples instinctively knew that nuts are best if soaked or sprouted before eaten. As with grains, raw and improperly prepared nuts contain several enzyme inhibitors that strain the digestive process. Mother Nature provides these inhibitors to delay the start of a nut's growth cycle until it is planted. However, if we soak nuts overnight in salt water (using Celtic sea salt), this process neutralizes the enzyme inhibitors, and the nuts become easier to digest. They can then be drained and dried gently in a warm oven or dehydrator for about 12 to 36 hours, until completely dry and crisp. We call them "crispy nuts." (See recipes in Chapter 9.)

Almonds, pecans, cashews, macadamia nuts and peanuts contain a high percentage of stable oleic acid, which does not go rancid quickly. These nuts can be stored in airtight containers at room temperature for many months. Walnuts, on the other hand, contain omega-3 linolenic acids, which is more susceptible to rancidity, and should always be stored in the refrigerator.

Although nuts are a nutritious food, if you have a digestive disorder of any kind, it is best to avoid them until you are completely healed.

CELTIC SEA SALT

Salt is a very important dietary component, and was used by virtually all traditional cultures. It provides sodium, which is a part of all body fluids and which regulates water balance, fluid distribution on both sides of cell membranes, muscle contraction and expansion, nerve stimulation and acid-alkaline balance. Additionally, sodium is vital to the proper functioning of the adrenal glands.

Salt also provides the most significant dietary source of chloride. Chloride is necessary for protein digestion, as it provides the chloride contained in hydrochloric acid. Salt also activates several enzymes needed for carbohydrate digestion. Additionally, salt is required for the development of the brain.

Unfortunately, most problems with salt are due to its processing. Few people realize that our salt is highly refined. The salt that you purchase in the grocery store is produced through a chemical and high-temperature industrial process that removes all the valuable magnesium salts as well as trace minerals. To keep salt dry, several additives are used, including aluminum compounds. To replace the natural iodine, potassium iodide is added, which is poorly absorbed and less effective than natural iodine in unrefined salt. To stabilize this iodide compound, dextrose is added, followed by a bleaching agent.

I make a point of using Celtic sea salt, which is extracted by the action of the sun on seawater in clay-lined vats. It is light gray in color, indicating a high moisture and trace mineral content. This salt contains about 82 percent sodium chloride, 14 percent macro-minerals, especially magnesium, and almost 80 trace minerals. It also provides a natural source of organic iodine, necessary for proper thyroid function.

CHEWING FOODS THOROUGHLY

Thoroughly chewing your foods before swallowing dramatically increases the assimilation of nutrients. This habit will aid in your recovery as you receive the highest benefit of a nutrient-dense diet.

## 6
# *SUPPLEMENTS*

*I*n addition to a diet of nutrient-dense foods, we recommend a few supplements to facilitate healing. To obtain these supplements, see Sources.

Note: You should consult with a holistic practitioner who works with traditional diets to determine your special supplement and dietary needs. Contact your local chapter of the Weston A. Price Foundation to find a practitioner who understands the Foundation's principles.

HIGH-VITAMIN COD LIVER OIL
AND HIGH-VITAMIN BUTTER OIL

In trying to provide his patients with ample amounts of fat-soluble vitamins A and D, necessary for the assimilation of proteins, minerals and water-soluble vitamins in foods, Dr. Price discovered the tremendous healing properties in the combination of high-vitamin butter oil and high-vitamin cod liver oil. With these two supplements, he was able to help his patients overcome osteoporosis, tooth decay, arthritis, rickets and failure to thrive in children. Other practitioners have subsequently found the combination to be excellent for digestive disorders. This therapy is an indispensable part of your recovery from digestive malfunction and inflammatory predisposition.

HIGH-VITAMIN COD LIVER OIL

Cod liver oil provides fat-soluble vitamins A and D, which Dr. Price found present in the diets of the healthy cultures he studied in amounts *ten* times higher than in the average American diet of his day. Cod liver oil also provides certain omega-3 fatty acids, called EPA and DHA, which in small amounts help to alleviate inflammatory tendencies.

High-vitamin cod liver oil is twice as concentrated as regular strength cod liver oil, so you don't need to take as much to obtain adequate amounts of vitamin A and D. As with all brands of cod liver oil imported into this country, high-vitamin cod liver oil is processed to remove all impurities.

We recommend one tablespoon of high-vitamin cod liver oil daily, or two tablespoons of regular strength, providing about 30,000 IU vitamin A and 3,000 IU vitamin D. This natural source of vitamins A and D is not toxic to the body, unlike synthetic versions found in supplements and pasteurized milk.

This supplement is best taken in the morning along with high-vitamin butter oil just before your other vitamin supplements and breakfast. It is easy to take by mixing it with a little water, and then swallowing fast. The brands we recommend do not have a strong fishy taste.

Note: Cod liver oil varies tremendously in quality. Please use the brands we recommend, as others may contain synthetics or the wrong proportions of vitamins A and D.

## 6. Supplements

HIGH VITAMIN BUTTER OIL

Dr. Price found that cod liver oil was much more effective when combined with high-vitamin butter oil. High-vitamin butter oil is made from the deep yellow butter that comes from cows feeding on rapidly growing grass in the spring and fall. The oil is centrifuged at a low temperature, which concentrates the nutrients in the oil.

High-vitamin butter oil supplies vitamins A and D, CLA (conjugated linoleic acid), the Wulzen Factor (called the "antistiffness" factor), anti-microbial butyric acid plus the X-Factor, a nutrient discovered by Dr. Price, which supports mineral metabolism. CLA in high-vitamin butter oil has been found to be a powerful anti-carcinogen. It also helps enhance muscle growth, lower insulin resistance and support the immune system. The Wulzen Factor, discovered by Dr. Rosalind Wulzen, helps promote flexibility in muscles, joints and tendons. It protects against calcification of the joints (degenerative arthritis), hardening of the arteries, cataracts and calcification of the pineal gland. Butyric acid is an important source of energy for cells of the gastrointestinal tract. It reduces inflammation of the intestinal wall and helps repair holes in the intestinal lining (leaky-gut syndrome). The X Factor is a powerful catalyst, which, like vitamins A and D, helps the body absorb and utilize minerals. (Note: These factors are also present in organ meats from grazing animals, egg yolks from pastured chickens and some seafood.)

We recommend one-half teaspoon butter oil daily in conjunction with high-vitamin cod liver oil (mixed with a little water), taken just before the morning meal.


ENZYME SUPPLEMENTS

If you consume lacto-fermented foods and beverages, you probably won't need an enzyme supplement. However, I found a superior enzyme supplement to be a great asset in helping my compromised digestive system break down foods completely, especially cooked foods.

Enzymes are not only necessary in the digestion of our foods, they also play a role in every process of the human body. (See books on enzymes by Dr. Edward Howell in Suggested Reading.) Without enzymes, we could not live. Enzymes contribute to every healing process that takes place in our cells, organs, tissues, muscles and tendons. We can enhance our body's own healing ability when we eat a diet high in enzymes and take additional enzymes supplements between meals. When exogenous enzymes are not taken with food, they add to the body's own enzyme resources.

The Radiant Life Company sells "Bioprime Pregest Cultured Enzymes," which provide excellent digestive support. I have found these enzymes to be extraordinary in effectiveness and reasonable in cost.

SBO-GREEN FOOD SUPPLEMENT

A product called "Super Greens and Dunaliella," by a company called Grainfields and available through the Radiant Life Company, combines a potent mixture of cereal grasses (gluten-free), micro-algae and kelp with a wide-spectrum, highly effective and hardy soil-based probiotic (SBO). Cereal grasses are high in chlorophyll, vitamins, protein, minerals and unique digestive enzymes. Micro-algae have significant amounts of lipid, protein, chlorophyll, carotenoid, vitamins, minerals and unique pigments. Kelp is considered the most completely mineralized food and is a particularly good source of iodine. This unique supplement will provide you with easy-to-digest nutrients and will help you build a healthy intestinal flora—the first step to healing the digestive system and building health.

I feel that this supplement is an outstanding partner to the fermented foods that I consume.

COLOSTRUM

Colostrum is the pre-milk fluid produced by all mammalian mothers for the first few days after giving birth—even people with milk allergies usually have no problem with it. Bovine colostrum contains immune growth factors virtually identical to those of humans. It can help accelerate healing of all tissues, including your intestinal tract, and build your immune system as it promotes the re-growth and re-colonization of beneficial bacteria in the bowel. Radiant Life offers a "first-milking colostrum" from grass-fed cows called "Immune Tree Colostrum."

VITAMIN AND MINERAL SUPPLEMENTS

To ensure that our nutritional requirements are met, vitamin and mineral supplements can be helpful when paired with a densely nutritious traditional diet. Our forefathers consumed *ten* to *fifty* times more vitamins, minerals and other nutrients than are supplied in our modern diets.

However, in choosing appropriate supplements you must consider the fact that most commercially available supplements—even those from health food stores—contain additives, such as magnesium stearate, which is used to speed up production. These additives cause the supplement to have a delayed absorption of nutrients, as they tend not to break down, or break down at the end of the digestive tract—past the area of ideal absorption. People with compromised digestion frequently have trouble utilizing the nutrients from these supplements and may develop allergic reactions. It is wise to avoid commercially produced supplements containing additives. Before I changed to additive-free supplements, all but one of the supplements I was taking contained magnesium stearate.

The following supplements are helpful for most people. It is best to take them just before the meal. (To order, see Sources.) A note of caution: Be wary of recommended supplement dosages, as they may be too high. Start supplements one at a time and if you notice any problems, cut back on the dosage.

- Multivitamin: A good additive-free multivitamin supplement is important in providing you with a wide array of nutrients necessary to building your health. "Doc's Best" vitamin, mineral and antioxidant supplement, developed by Dr. Ron Schmid, is an example of a superior additive-free multivitamin.
- Calcium/magnesium: Calcium is the most prevalent mineral in

the body, and adequate calcium absorption is an important key to good health. Without calcium, the body cannot function properly. Vital not only for strong bones and teeth, calcium is also needed for heart and muscle function, nervous system and acid-alkaline balance. The best food sources of calcium are bone broths and raw dairy products, but along with these foods, a good calcium supplement can help you recover from a depleted state and help maintain sufficient calcium levels. Calcium should be taken in conjunction with magnesium. Most calcium/magnesium supplements are difficult to absorb. However microcrystalline hydroxyapatite concentrate (MCHC) is the finest source of bio-available calcium. A note of caution: Taking too much calcium/magnesium supplement may cause loose stools. Cut back on the dosage if you experience this problem.

- Vitamin E: Vitamin E is a critical fat-soluble antioxidant that is needed for circulation, tissue repair and healing. It seems to retard the aging process because it helps to deactivate free radicals. The best available vitamin E supplement is called "Unique E." It is a natural vitamin E complex made without soybean oil. Soybean oil is found in most Vitamin E supplements and can become rancid, thereby altering its antioxidant properties.

- Vitamin C: Vitamin C, a water-soluble vitamin, is needed for a multitude of processes including tissue growth and repair, strength of capillary walls and adrenal function. It promotes healing of wounds and is a powerful antioxidant.

# 7
# MAKING IT PRACTICAL

**M**usicians' lives are filled with complex schedules—every day can be different. In our professional schedule, we juggle practicing, rehearsal schedules, concerts, teaching, travel and—our favorite subject—*traffic!* Athletes, dancers and people in other fields experience comparable complications. In our private lives, all of us coordinate family time and schedules, exercise, personal needs, health care, shopping, cooking, cleaning, lawn care, hobbies. . . the list goes on! Most feel blessed to have creative lives in an interesting and challenging field.

What we need most is *energy—vibrant energy!* When we feel our *spark*, we meet our daily complexities with joy and ease. When we do not feel well, our complex schedule can turn into a complex *burden.* In every respect, a whole-foods, traditional diet can help support our energy requirements and correct health issues that may challenge our career.

But how can we practically incorporate a diet rich in traditional foods when many times we are gone for the entire day?

The first requirement is a firm commitment to health—long-term vibrant health. Musicians, athletes and dancers develop something early on that many people struggle to achieve—that is *discipline*. If we are able to have the discipline required to become professionals, we certainly can acquire the discipline and planning required to support the health of our bodies. However, we are certainly not the only people who can generate the discipline required to make crucial changes. When you feel the increase in energy that comes from an enzyme-rich, nutrient-dense diet and begin solving your health problems through this approach, you will find that you crave only foods that nourish your body and have no desire to return to processed or refined foods—*you* are worth the effort!

Planning is the key to healthy eating away from home. A few items can allow you to bring an entire day's worth of food for your demanding schedule. You can find these items reasonably priced at almost any department store. They are:

- A large thermal insulated bag
- Several large thermoses for hot foods and drinks
- Leak-proof food and drink containers for cold foods and fermented beverages
- Ice packs for cold foods

Once a commitment is made, locating a good supply of meat, milk products and eggs from pasture-raised animals is key. A good place to start is the nearest local chapter of the Weston A. Price Foundation, which can be found at the website, www.WestonAPrice.org, by calling (202) 333-363-4394, or by e-mail (info@westonaprice.org).

You will need to implement a new way of shopping for your high-quality animal foods. I order my foods from a farm cooperative one week in advance and pick them up the following week—this is the procedure for the co-op that brings the food to my area. I actually find this to be very efficient. When I go to pick up my food, it is ready for me to put in my car. I am literally done "shopping" in five to ten minutes and on my way home. It is also great to have such a direct relationship to the farmers who are producing the foods that I eat. They truly care about the people in their co-op and have become good friends. The rest of my food, which is mostly produce, I pick up at the health food store.

You will also want to spend about one-half day a week doing some advance cooking and food preparation so that meals will be easy to put together. During this period devoted to food prep you will:

- Start a soup stock (beef, chicken or fish)
- Prepare lacto-fermented dairy foods (yogurt, kefir, or cultured cream)
- Prepare other fermented beverages and foods such as coconut kefir and yogurt, beet kvass, and sauerkraut
- Start a batch of crispy nuts
- Make a large batch of soup or stew from a stock prepared earlier

You can build easy travel meals by selecting from some of these very portable foods. Some of the easiest options are:

- Alternating a variety of soups made from broths
- Kefir and yogurt—made either from raw milk or young coconuts
- Smoothies made from raw milk or coconut kefir or yogurt
- A thermos of warm coconut milk tonic or raw milk tonic
- A thermos of herbal or green tea with cream or whole coconut milk
- Raw milk cheese—from cows or goats
- Crispy nuts
- Salads made with leftover chicken, fish or beef and vegetables
- Smoked salmon or trout
- Paté or liverwurst
- Other leftovers

Although it is tempting to eat from vending machines or purchase fast food, your commitment to your own health is worth the trouble of finding ways to eat foods that will *consistently* provide you with the highest possible benefit—remember, every meal and snack counts! I often picture myself eating like someone from one of the healthy populations that Dr. Price studied—as if I had gone back in time to an era when foods were of a completely different quality.

With these goals in mind, we recommend that eating in restaurants should, in general, be limited. While some restaurant foods may be well prepared, food quality is, at best, questionable. Most restaurants buy foods that are substandard and use seasonings containing MSG. Fast food restaurants should be strictly avoided. If you have no other choice, eat at the highest quality restaurant that you can afford, order simple foods that need little preparation, and make sure to specify that your food is cooked with traditional fats such as olive oil or pure butter.

If you are gluten sensitive, beware of hidden gluten contamination such as a griddle that is dually used to toast bread and cook meats, or "broiled" fish that is lightly dusted with flour so it won't stick to the grill. (This happened to me even though I had specified that I could have no flour. Before I noticed the thin film of flour on my fish, I had eaten several bites, and I was sick for many days after.) In fact, the Celiac Foundation suggests that it may be helpful to print a small, discreet card that says something like, "I have celiac disease and cannot eat any foods containing gluten—wheat, rye, oats or barley, or seasonings with barley malt, MSG and soy sauce. If I eat even a small amount of these foods or seasonings, I may become seriously ill. Thank you for your help."

For your driving trips, take a large cooler packed with the foods that you will need. If you are traveling by air, good quality raw cheese, crispy nuts, canned sardines in water or olive oil and canned tuna will do in a pinch. (Purchase your tuna from the health food store—commercial brands of tuna from the regular grocery store *always* contain MSG.)

# 7. Making It Practical

Changes to routine can be difficult to make. Rather than attempt climbing the entire mountain in one day, take small steps and gradually add nutrient-dense foods to your diet. Once you experience the good results, you will be inspired to add more healing foods. Try these small steps to get started:

- Purchase a high quality cod-liver oil: we recommend 1 tablespoon daily (see Sources). Cod liver oil is easy to take mixed with a little water and swallowed quickly.
- Add saturated fats such as organic butter and coconut oil to your diet.
- Make one cultured food such as sauerkraut and consume with meals containing cooked foods (see Chapter 9).
- Make some crispy nuts; they're very easy to prepare (see Chapter 9).
- Make a bone broth soup (see Chapter 9) and consume daily.
- While locating a source for raw milk, purchase a high-quality, organic plain *whole* milk yogurt such as Traderspoint, Brown Cow, Seven Stars or Stoneyfield, and make one smoothie daily (see Chapter 9) or eat plain with berries (don't forget to add 2-3 raw, organic, free-range egg yolks to your smoothie).
- Have plain whole yogurt and berries, or crispy nuts and organic cheese, for a snack instead of low-nutrient snacks.
- Cut out sugar, vegetable oils (except olive oil and sesame seed oil), grains and any processed foods from your diet and replace with nutrient-dense foods.
- Use Celtic sea salt (see Sources) instead of refined salt.

In the following detailed menu plan, try to incorporate as many components as you can. If you have a serious digestive disorder such as chronic diarrhea or constipation, IBS, Celiac or Crohn's, begin by consuming bone broths and blended bone-broth soups exclusively until your digestive system is calm and then add other foods. *Restoring*

*Your Digestive Health,* by Jordan Rubin and Joseph Brasco, contains an excellent protocol for healing an inflamed digestive tract.

SIX-DAY HEALING MENU

Your healing diet should include:
  + High quality proteins at every meal (prepared rare, to keep enzymes intact, or gently cooked in broth)
  + Ample traditional fats—raw butter or coconut oil with foods at every meal
  + Fermented beverages and foods daily
  + Organ meats at least twice a week
  + Bone broths daily
  + Highly nutritious snacks such as raw milk or coconut kefir, crispy nuts, and raw milk cheese from cows or goats
  + One raw salad daily if your digestion system is healed
  + A variety of cooked vegetables with butter, lard or coconut oil
  + Low-sugar fruit in strict moderation
  + Celtic sea salt in place of other kinds of salt

Along with your daily menu, be sure to include your supplements. These are best taken just before you eat, except for the SBO supplement, which is best taken on an empty stomach:

  + High-vitamin cod liver oil
  + High-vitamin butter oil
  + SBO Super Greens supplement
  + Perfect Food Supplement with coconut oil (to absorb nutrients in supplement)
  + Digestive enzymes (with cooked foods)
  + Other supplements that are appropriate for you

You should not feel hungry with this diet because it will provide ample fats (which maintain blood sugar levels), adequate protein and nutrient density.

# 7. Making It Practical

We are also recommending eating unheated raw butter from grass-fed cows at every meal. It is an extremely important dietary element that can be added to each meal, and it will be a tremendous aid in your healing. It is delicious not only on vegetables, but also on meat and fish. It is the number one health food, as it provides vitamins A and D, the catalyst for nutrient absorption and many factors that help heal the intestinal lining. Raw butter was a key element in my recovery.

Recipes for these menus are included in Chapter 9.

## DAY ONE

### UPON RISING
- 1 cup beet kvass mixed with SBO Super Greens supplement (see Sources)
- 1-2 tablespoons coconut oil melted in warm water or herb tea

### BREAKFAST
- Supplements (1 tablespoon high-vitamin cod liver oil, 1/2 teaspoon high-vitamin butter oil and other supplements appropriate for you)
- Raw milk kefir or yogurt smoothie
  OR
- Young coconut kefir with coconut yogurt or creamed coconut smoothie

### LUNCH
- Supplements
- Raw milk or homemade ginger ale
- Meat, fish or poultry
- Salad of fresh greens and assorted raw vegetables with homemade dressing (only if your digestive system is healed)
  OR
- Steamed vegetables with raw butter

SNACK
- Kefir or coconut milk tonic or raw milk tonic
- Gluten-free nut crackers with butter

DINNER
- Supplements
- Raw milk or homemade ginger ale
- Chicken soup
- Lamb chop, rare, sautéed in butter or lard, served with raw butter
- Steamed broccoli with raw butter

### DAY TWO

UPON RISING
- 1 cup beet kvass mixed with SBO Super Green supplement (see Sources)
- 1-2 tablespoons coconut oil melted in warm water

BREAKFAST
- Supplements (1 tablespoon high-vitamin cod liver oil, 1/2 teaspoon high-vitamin butter oil and other supplements appropriate for you)
- Kefir, raw milk or coconut kefir
- Two or three eggs sautéed in butter, sunny side up
- Bacon (no nitrate)

LUNCH
- Supplements
- Raw milk or homemade ginger ale
- Beef liver, rare, sautéed in butter or coconut oil, served with raw butter
- Onions and beet greens sautéed in butter or coconut oil
- Fresh raw sauerkraut

# 7. Making It Practical

SNACK
- Plain yogurt, coconut milk tonic or raw milk tonic and crispy nuts

DINNER
- Supplements
- Raw milk or homemade ginger ale
- Chicken soup (leftover) with cream (optional)
- Small ribeye steak, rare, sautéed in butter or coconut oil, served with raw butter
- Steamed spinach with raw butter
  OR
- Salad of fresh greens and vegetables with homemade dressing (only if your digestive system is healed)

## DAY THREE

UPON RISING
- 1 cup beet kvass mixed with SBO Super Green supplement (see Sources)
- 1-2 tablespoons coconut oil melted in warm water

BREAKFAST
- Supplements (1 tablespoon high-vitamin cod liver oil, 1/2 teaspoon high-vitamin butter oil and other supplements appropriate for you)
- Raw milk yogurt or coconut yogurt
- Fresh raspberries
- Superscramble

LUNCH
- Supplements
- Raw milk kefir, raw milk or homemade ginger ale
- Chicken soup (leftover)
- Steamed broccoli with raw butter

SNACK
- Raw milk kefir or coconut milk tonic or raw milk tonic and crispy nuts

DINNER
- Supplements
- Raw milk or homemade ginger ale
- Wild caught salmon sautéed or baked in butter or coconut oil
- Parsnips and carrots sautéed in butter or coconut oil, served with raw butter
- Fresh raw sauerkraut

### DAY FOUR

UPON RISING
- 1 cup beet kvass mixed with SBO Super Green supplement (see Sources)
- 1-2 tablespoons coconut oil melted in warm water

BREAKFAST
- Supplements (1 tablespoon high-vitamin cod liver oil, 1/2 teaspoon high-vitamin butter oil and other supplements appropriate for you)
- Raw milk or coconut kefir
- Steak cooked rare, sautéed in butter or coconut oil
- Blueberries and fresh cream, creamed coconut or coconut milk

LUNCH
- Supplements
- Raw milk or homemade ginger ale
- Sardines with a fresh salad of greens and vegetables with homemade dressing (only if your digestive system is healed)
  OR
- Canned wild salmon with steamed green beans and raw butter

SNACK
- Raw milk kefir, coconut milk tonic or raw milk tonic
- Gluten-free nut crackers with butter

DINNER
- Supplements
- Raw milk or coconut kefir
- Beef-vegetable soup
- Steamed Swiss chard with raw butter

## DAY FIVE

UPON RISING
- 1 cup beet kvass mixed with SBO Super Green supplement (see Sources)
- 1-2 tablespoons coconut oil melted in warm water

BREAKFAST
- Supplements (1 tablespoon high-vitamin cod liver oil, 1/2 teaspoon high-vitamin butter oil and other supplements appropriate for you)
- Raw milk or coconut kefir
- Omelet with raw cow or goat cheese and vegetables
- Bacon (no nitrate) or scrapple (no additives)

LUNCH
- Supplements
- Raw milk or homemade ginger ale
- Chicken liver paté on celery sticks or coconut crackers or gluten-free nut crackers
- Steamed broccoli with raw butter

SNACK
Raw milk yogurt or coconut yogurt with blueberries

DINNER
- Supplements
- Raw milk or homemade ginger ale
- Ground beef heart and ground beef entrée
- Steamed carrots and peas with raw butter
- Fresh raw sauerkraut

### DAY SIX

UPON RISING
- 1 cup beet kvass mixed with SBO Super Green supplement (see Sources)
- 1-2 tablespoons coconut oil melted in warm water

BREAKFAST
- Supplements (1 tablespoon high-vitamin cod liver oil, 1/2 teaspoon high-vitamin butter oil and other supplements appropriate for you)
- 2-3 eggs sautéed in butter or coconut oil—sunny side up
- Bacon (no nitrate)
- Raw milk or coconut yogurt with fruit

LUNCH
- Supplements
- Raw milk or coconut kefir
- Beef-vegetable soup (leftover)
- Baked butternut squash with raw butter

SNACK
- Raw cow or goat cheese

DINNER
- Supplements
- Raw milk or homemade ginger ale
- Wild caught shrimp sautéed in butter or coconut oil or in whole coconut milk
- Steamed broccoli with raw butter
- Baked butternut squash with raw butter

*8*

# SUGGESTED READING

I strongly encourage you to continue your healing journey by seeking out detailed information. As you heal, you will in turn help others—you are not alone in pain by any means. Having in-depth knowledge will give you the necessary insight to be a light for others.

First, please investigate the Weston A. Price Foundation's website at www.westonaprice.org. There is a wealth of information to guide you in this incredible resource. Become a member and receive the foundations quarterly magazine.

The following books are highly recommended:

*Nutrition and Physical Degeneration*
by Weston A. Price, DDS
Published by Price-Pottenger Nutrition Foundation

An astounding masterpiece, Dr. Weston Price's work describes the advent of chronic illness and degenerative conditions in traditional populations that adopted Western denatured foods, and describes the dietary principles of fourteen isolated cultures worldwide who for thousands of years were immune to these degenerative conditions. His research has fueled a growing movement of people dedicated to healing through consuming traditional foods and supporting the return of small family farms that follow traditional methods. Available through the Radiant Life Wellness Catalog, radiantlifecatalog.com, and amazon.com

*Nourishing Traditions: The Cookbook that Challenges Politically Correct Nutrition and the Diet Dictocrats*
By Sally Fallon and Mary G. Enig, PhD
Published by NewTrends Publishing

Sally Fallon presents us with a unique cookbook of traditional healthful and timeless recipes that have sustained cultures worldwide, with an important introductory section that discusses the problems with today's health trends and guides you to the necessary elements of optimal and sustaining nutrition. The founder of the Weston A. Price Foundation and an international lecturer, Sally Fallon is truly an inspiration. Her book will be a tremendous partner in your healing quest.

*The Untold Story of Milk*
By Ron Schmid, ND
Published by NewTrends Publishing

Dr. Schmid thoroughly explores the amazing history of milk as an important element of people's diets worldwide, as a cure for chronic illnesses of all kinds and as a commodity that sustains traditional cultures. He traces milk's terrible decline in quality due to abuses in the dairy industry beginning in the 1800s. He gives light to the complex problems that compulsory pasteurization has caused, not only to people's health, but to the very economic structures of our society, now controlled by governmental regulation and the factory farming industry. He gives solutions to these issues by offering accurate information on the incredible health and economic merits of again supporting a healthful supply of clean, raw milk in our country.

*Patient Heal Thyself*
By Jordan S. Rubin,  NMD, CNC
Published by Freedom Press

Dr. Rubin's book unlocked the first door to my recovery. His terrifying illness and path to vibrant health helped me to understand basic information about digestive illnesses and how to begin to approach my healing. His leadership is helping thousands of people find the tools they require to overcome the multitudes of chronic illnesses that are affecting so many people in our country.

(Note: In both this book and the next listed, Rubin puts a high emphasis on the healing properties of goat's milk yogurt, but only briefly mentions the merits of raw milk from pastured cows, while correctly criticizing pasteurized milk. For most people, raw milk from cows on pasture offers the same healing benefits as does raw goat's milk, and raw cow's milk is more readily available.)

*Restoring Your Digestive Health*
By Jordan S. Rubin, NMD, CNC, and Joseph Brasco, MD
Published by Twin Streams Health

Another important resource that can help you correct and overcome any kind of digestive disorder. Jordan Rubin and Dr. Brasco have helped countless individuals find solutions to digestive disorders. The protocols in this book for treating digestive problems have successfully helped thousands of patients. I highly recommend this book if you have any digestive complaints. It may help you "cut to the chase" and save you ineffective medical care that may not solve your underlying problems. (See note in previous review.)

*Enzyme Nutrition*
By Edward Howell, MD
Published by Avery

Enzymes control every mechanism in your body. Without enzymes, life is not possible. Each of us has an enzyme bank or "potential," which, if used up, will cause our bodies to deteriorate. Dr. Howell, who was one of the world's foremost experts on enzyme research and who lived past one hundred years, teaches us about the necessity of eating enzyme-rich foods—especially raw animal foods such as raw milk, raw or lightly cooked meats or raw egg yolks—that do not cause us to use up our enzyme potential. (Only high-quality, traditionally raised animal foods can be safely eaten in this raw state.) This was also one of the important practices amongst the healthy populations.

Howell discusses the fact that digestive enzymes should be present in our foods, as in raw foods, or be taken with foods, as in enzyme supplements, to save our body's enzymes for the necessary functions of energy production and repair. In *Enzyme Nutrition,* he covers a wealth of significant research on enzymes and describes their importance in maximizing life expectancy.

However, Dr. Howell, an avid promoter of raw foods, does not cover the enzyme benefits of fermented foods and beverages—a worldwide practice for millennia. Through eating fermented foods, we have another endless supply of enzymes available in conjunction with those present in raw foods.

As a high-enzyme diet is critical to optimal health, it is clearly beneficial to artists and athletes and those whose work requires the repetitive use of the same muscle groups. Howell points out that when we often eat foods devoid of enzymes, such as refined or processed foods and cooked foods without accompanying fermented foods, our body is forced to spend a lot of energy on producing digestive enzymes.

When our body must continually produce digestive enzymes, the enzymes that are intended for maintenance and repair will be sacrificed. The longer this process goes on, the quicker degenerative conditions, such as inflammatory responses, will develop. Therefore, a diet high in enzyme-rich foods, such as raw animal foods and fermented foods, ensures that our body's vital enzymes will be available for supporting optimal physiological function.

*Enzymes for Health and Longevity*
By Edward Howell, MD
Published by Avery

Dr. Howell's second book is another exciting journal of research on the effects of high-enzyme diets on longevity. This is a fascinating book that will further your understanding of this very important subject.

*Fiber Menace*
By Konstantin Monastyrsky
Published by Ageless Press

*Fiber Menace* describes major health problems that can develop from eating what's considered a modern healthy diet high in fiber from grains, vegetables, fruits, legumes and even fiber supplements. The author details how high-fiber diets cause large stools which stretch the intestinal tract beyond its normal range—eventually resulting in intestinal damage—and a drastic upset of the natural bacterial flora of the gut. The end results manifest as hernias, hemorrhoidal disease, constipation, malnourishment, irritable bowel syndrome and Crohn's disease. He also provides numerous medical references to show that high-fiber diets do not confer the benefits claimed for them. One fascinating chapter of Monastyrsky's book details the problems with drinking too much water.

*The Cholesterol Myths: Exposing the Fallacy*
*that Saturated Fat and Cholesterol Cause Heart Disease*
Uffe Ravnskov, MD, PhD
Published by New Tends Publishing, 2000)

This is an important book for those whose fear of cholesterol and saturated fat prevents them from embracing the principles of traditional diets, rich in fat and cholesterol. Dr. Ravnskov clearly shows how the research cited to "prove" that cholesterol and saturated fat cause heart disease is severely flawed and in many cases falsified. Ravnskov presents the many technical studies in highly readable and often humorous form. An excellent book for laymen to read. . . and then give to their doctors.

*Pasture Perfect*
By Jo Robinson
Published by Vashon Island Press

An eye-opening and often shocking book that compares the enormous nutritional differences between meats, dairy, eggs and poultry from animals traditionally raised on pasture to those coming from the industrial farming model. Robinson also gives us an accurate first-hand look at the many unfortunate practices of corporate agribusiness, which has forced out small family farms, drastically diminished the quality of animals' health, degraded our food supply and our health and caused continuous harm to our environment.

The author presents solutions by pointing to the large movement of farmers who have pulled out of the destructive corporate farming system and are reaping the vast benefits, joined by those who are returning to the superior, ecologically sound methods of traditional grass farming. As these farmers are producing extraordinarily healthful foods that are quickly growing in demand by a public searching for nutritional answers to healing chronic illness, they are also receiving direct and well-deserved financial reward for their much-needed service.

*The Fourfold Path to Healing*
By Thomas S. Cowan, MD
Published by NewTrends Publishing

Dr. Cowan merges the wisdom of traditional societies, the most modern findings of Western medicine and the esoteric teachings of the ancients as he answers this important question: "How do we obtain true health?" *The Fourfold Path to Healing* is a unique, comprehensive view that will challenge your deepest beliefs while showing you a practical approach to healing. Includes chapters devoted to the fifteen most common disease conditions.

*Eat Fat Lose Fat*
By Mary G. Enig, PhD and Sally Fallon
Published by Hudson Street Press

The healthy alternative to *trans* fats, this revolutionary program explains why we must eat healthy, saturated fats—especially coconut oil—to achieve weight loss and good health.

Since the late 1950s, it's been drilled into Americans that fat makes you fat, saturated fats (such as those found in butter, eggs and red meat) are unhealthy, and tropical fats and oils (like coconut and palm) are downright deadly. And yet—as we eliminate saturated fats from our diet for fear of high cholesterol levels and hardened arteries—obesity, heart disease and cancer rates have continued to climb.

Based on more than two decades of research by world-renowned biochemist and fats expert Dr. Mary Enig, *Eat Fat, Lose Fat* flouts conventional wisdom by explaining why vegetable oils (such as soybean and corn oils) are in large part responsible for our national obesity and health crises, while the saturated fats currently considered "harmful" are, in fact, essential to weight loss and good overall health.

World populations on four continents that subsist on the coconut, with less evidence of heart disease, weight gain or other chronic illnesses, provide the best proof of this food's safety and efficacy; dozens of studies conducted by prestigious, mainstream universities support the use of coconut and other healthy fats and reveal the faulty reasoning underlying the saturated fat/heart disease hypothesis; and case stories from a wide range of people illustrate how using coconut oil in concert with other healthy fats can spark weight loss and heal serious chronic illness, including anxiety, hypothyroidism and chronic fatigue syndrome.

Featuring delicious recipes for each of its three nutritional programs, *Eat Fat, Lose Fat* is the book to help you build energy, lose weight, fight disease, and boost your immunity.


*Dangerous Grains*
By James Braly, MD and Ron Hogan
Published by Avery

*Dangerous Grains* will give you an introduction to the health problems associated with gluten sensitivity and celiac disease. This book documents the rapidly growing percentage of people who have trouble digesting and tolerating grains.

# 8. Suggested Reading

*Know Your Fats*
Mary G. Enig, PhD
Published by Bethseda Press

Dr. Enig is one of the world's leading experts in fat and lipid research. This primer will give you accurate and useful background on the complicated subject of fats and oils. The book highlights the importance of traditional fats for our health and will help you understand the devastating problems caused by vegetable oils and *trans* fats that flooded our food supply after the Second World War.

*The Inflammation Syndrome*
By Jack Challem
Published by Wiley

Challem, a leading health and medical writer, has offered another resource for dealing with inflammation tendencies. He is not a proponent of raw milk, but offers another look at dietary influences on a predisposition to inflammation and further information on primitive diets and problems with our food supply.

## 9
# RECIPES

*H*ere are a few basic recipes to get you started, many of which are taken from *Nourishing Traditions,* by my co-author, Sally Fallon. We suggest that you also look at the wealth of other wonderful recipes contained in *Nourishing Traditions* to add variety and interest to your meals. Happy health and cooking!

### CULTURED DAIRY PRODUCTS

Included here are a few recipes for cultured dairy products. Although we have presented them using fresh raw milk, it is possible to make them from commercial milk—though not as healthful. For kefir, you will want to follow the special instructions on the starter package for commercial milk.

Kefir is a wonderful, health promoting, easy-to-make beverage. It is very portable and is great for breakfast and snacks. Kefir is a high-enzyme, nutrient-dense food that helps restore and maintain the inner intestinal ecology. I always take kefir on days away from home. I make a gallon at a time, saving a cup at the end to make my next batch. The first step to kefir is preparing a starter batch. You will need resealable glass or stainless steel containers.

There are several ways to make kefir. It can be made with kefir grains or with kefir powder. This recipe is made with kefir powder.

KEFIR STARTER
Makes 1 quart

> *1 package kefir powder (see Sources)*
> *1 quart fresh whole raw milk*

In a glass jar or stainless steel container, stir the kefir powder into the milk. You needn't heat the milk, as the directions on the package may suggest. Heating is not necessary with raw milk. Cover the jar. Place in a warm place that has a temperature of 65 to 76 degrees (such as on top of your refrigerator), for 18 to 24 hours until it achieves the tartness of your liking. Now you are ready to make a larger batch. If the kefir ferments too long, it will separate—not to worry, see recipe below for kefir cheese and whey. Enjoy the kefir cheese and use the whey to ferment other foods and beverages.

KEFIR
Makes 1 gallon

> *1 gallon fresh whole raw milk*
> *1 cup kefir starter*

Pour the gallon of milk into a wide-mouth glass jar or stainless steel container. Stir in the starter and cover. Place in a warm place (65 to 76 degrees). The kefir will be ready in 18 to 24 hours. Of course, you can make smaller amounts if you like—you will go through kefir quickly if you are drinking a quart a day.

# 9. Recipes

KEFIR SMOOTHIE
Makes about 2 1/2 cups

*2 cups kefir*
*2-4 raw egg yolks (discard the egg white*
  *or save to make into macaroons)*
*1 tablespoon extra virgin coconut oil (optional)*
*1/2-1 cup berries*
*1 tablespoon raw honey (optional)*

Blend ingredients and enjoy as a quick breakfast or snack.

KEFIR CHEESE AND WHEY
Makes 5 cups whey and 3 cups kefir cheese

*2 quarts raw whole milk*
*1/2 cup kefir starter*

Lacto-fermented recipes call for whey as a starter culture. The cream cheese, which is a by-product, is far superior to the commercial variety.

Put the milk and kefir starter in a wide-mouth glass jar. Let the kefir ferment until it visibly separates into white curds and yellowish whey. This will take 1 to 4 days. Line a large strainer set over a bowl with a clean non-terry cloth dishtowel. Pour in the separated milk, cover and let stand at room temperature for several hours. The whey will run into the bowl, and the milk solids will stay in the strainer. Tie up the towel with the milk solids inside, being careful not to squeeze. Tie this little sack to a wooden spoon placed across a deep container so that more whey can drip out. When the bag stops dripping, the cheese is ready. Store whey in a mason jar and cream cheese in a covered glass container. Refrigerated, the cream cheese keeps for about 3 weeks and the whey for about 6 months.

Variation: Easy Whey

Use *1 quarts plain whole yoghurt* (recipe below or see Sources) instead of separated raw milk. Makes 2 1/2 cups whey and 1 1/2 cups cream cheese.

RAW MILK YOGURT
Makes 1 quart

> *3 tablespoons plus 2 teaspoons good quality*
> *commercial plain yogurt (see Sources) or yogurt from previous batch*
> *1 quart fresh whole raw milk*

Place milk in a double boiler and heat to 110 degrees. Remove 2 teaspoons of warm milk and add 1 tablespoon yogurt. Stir well and pour into a quart-sized wide-mouth mason jar. Add a further 2 tablespoons plus 2 teaspoons yogurt to the jar and stir well. Cover tightly and place in a large pot along with a hot water bottle. Cover the pot. Let sit for about eight hours. Transfer to the refrigerator.

You can also make whey and cream cheese out of your yogurt. Drain the yogurt through a large strainer lined with a non-terry cloth dish towel. Follow directions for kefir cheese and whey.

Note: If using commercial milk—gently heat the whole milk to 180 degrees and allow to cool to about 110 degrees. Stir in ½ cup yogurt and place in a warm oven (about 150 degrees) overnight. In the morning transfer to the refrigerator. (Throughout the day, use paper towels to mop up any whey that exudes from the yogurt.)

YOGURT SMOOTHIE
Makes about 2 1/2 cups

> *2 cups yogurt*
> *2-4 raw egg yolks (discard the egg white or*
> *save to make into macaroons)*
> *1 tablespoon extra virgin coconut oil (optional)*

# 9. Recipes

*1/2-1 cup berries*
*1 tablespoon raw honey (optional)*

Blend ingredients and enjoy for breakfast or as a snack.

RAW MILK TONIC
Makes 2 cups

*1 1/2 cups whole, certified clean raw milk, at room temperature*
*1/4 cup cream, not ultrapasteurized*
*2 tablespoons molasses*
*2-4 egg yolks*
*1/2 teaspoon vanilla extract*
  *(if gluten sensitive, use alcohol-free; see Sources)*

Blend ingredients together with a whisk. May be heated gently to about 90 degrees.

COCONUT RECIPES

COCONUT MILK TONIC
Makes about 1 quart

*1 can whole organic coconut milk (preferably organic)*
*1 1/2 cups water*
*1 tablespoon maple syrup or other natural sweetener (or to taste)*
*1/2 teaspoon vanilla or almond extract*
  *(if gluten sensitive, use alcohol-free; see Sources)*
*1 teaspoon dolomite powder (calcium carbonate; see Sources)*
*1/2 teaspoon cinnamon (optional)*

Warm gently. This is a good substitute for raw milk. It is great to take to work in a thermos. It contains the same calories, fat and calcium as raw milk.

CULTURED YOUNG COCONUT PRODUCTS

If you have tried fresh raw milk kefir and plain raw milk from pastured cows and have an allergic response such as diarrhea, you may be intolerant to even high quality dairy. This is quite unusual as most people who are lactose intolerant do extremely well on raw milk and raw milk products. If you are one of the few people who experience difficulties with raw milk, coconut kefir and yogurt cultured from young coconuts is a delicious, densely nutritious alternative.

Coconut products have been a traditional health-building food for millennia. Cultured coconut beverages and foods aid in digestion, as they help to build your intestinal flora. They are high in valuable minerals, including potassium, iodine, calcium and magnesium. The pudding-like meat in these coconuts is high in protein, is enzyme rich, and serves as an excellent source of lauric and caprylic acid, which aid in the healing of the digestive system. Finally, coconut kefir has a beneficial cleansing effect on the endocrine system. (Note: If substituting coconut kefir for raw milk kefir, be sure to eat plenty of organ meats, egg yolks, and bone broth soups to ensure that you consume the dense nutrition you will require when you aren't able to consume dairy. A good source of raw goat's milk and milk products from pastured goats is also worth investigating, as many people who cannot tolerate cow's milk do fine on goat's milk.)

COCONUT KEFIR AND YOGURT
Makes 1 quart

> *3 young coconuts*
> *kefir starter powder (see Sources)*

Empty coconut water from young coconuts by first shaving a few layers from the bottom of the coconut until a circle appears. Keep on shaving until two more circles appear. Take a sharp object and poke through the biggest hole. Pour the clear liquid into a glass jar and stir in the kefir starter powder. (Note: If liquid is pink, do not use—it is spoiled.) Let the liquid sit on the counter 18-24 hours. It is done when the color changes to milky white and there is a bit of bubbling on the top. This means that all the sugar has been transformed. The kefir will taste pleasantly tart. Transfer to the refrigerator. Coconut kefir will last for about three weeks.

To enjoy the coconut meat inside, you can eat it as is or enhance its nutrient value by making it into *coconut yogurt.* To open the coconut, place a meat cleaver across the diameter of the coconut and pound it partially through the coconut with a large, hard plastic hammer. After the coconut is penetrated, pound the cleaver at the overhanging end until coconut is split—do this *outside!* Scoop the meat out. The meat should be a bright white—if it is translucent, it should be discarded. Make yogurt by processing the meat with a blender or food processor until smooth and culturing with either 1/4 cup of previously made coconut kefir or 1 package of kefir starter powder. Stir either the coconut kefir or kefir starter powder into the processed coconut meat and leave mixture at room temperature 12-18 hours. It will taste slightly tart and can be eaten plain or used in smoothies. Transfer to refrigerator.

Save 1/2 cup of coconut kefir for making your next quart of kefir and yogurt. If making larger quantities, proportionately more kefir is needed as a starter. (I culture an entire gallon of kefir at a time with a case of coconuts. This requires 1 cup of starter.)

(Note: Coconut kefir can be used to prepare other cultured beverages and foods in place of whey if you have allergies to milk.)

CULTURED COCONUT SMOOTHIE
Serves 1

> *1 cup coconut kefir*
> *1/2-3/4 cup coconut yogurt, blended coconut meat, whole coconut milk*
>     *or 2 tablespoons creamed coconut dissolved in ¼ cup warm water*
> *3-4 egg yolks*
> *1 cup berries (optional)*
> *1-2 tablespoons raw honey (optional)*

Blend all ingredients until smooth.

## FERMENTED BEVERAGES

Fermented beverages are the perfect healthy alternative to soft drinks; they give the body a lift by providing nutrients in a form that is quickly assimilated, rather than by stimulating the adrenal glands with sugar and caffeine.

We have provided two recipes here. (There are many more in *Nourishing Traditions*, by Sally Fallon.) Beet Kvass is a medicinal drink especially good for candida, usually taken morning and evening. Ginger Ale is delicious and refreshing with meals.

BEET KVASS
Makes 2 quarts

> *3 medium or 2 large organic beets, peeled and chopped up coarsely*
> *1/4 cup homemade whey (pages 107-108) or 1/4 cup coconut kefir*
> *1/4 cup fresh ginger (optional), finely chopped*
> *1 tablespoon Celtic sea salt (see Sources)*
> *filtered water*

This drink is valuable for its medicinal qualities and as a digestive aid. Beets are just loaded with nutrients. One 4-ounce glass, morning and night, is an excellent blood tonic, promotes regularity, aids digestion, alkalizes the blood, cleanses the liver and is a good treatment for kidney stones and other ailments. Beet kvass may be also be used in place of vinegar in salad dressings and as an addition to soups.

Place beets, whey and salt in a 2-quart glass container. Add filtered water to fill the container. Stir well and cover securely. Keep at room temperature for 2 days before transferring to the refrigerator.

When most of the liquid has been drunk, you may fill up the container with water and keep at room temperature for another two days. The resulting brew will be less strong than the first. After the second brew, discard the beets and start again. You may, however, reserve some of the liquid and use this as your inoculant instead of whey.

Note: Do not use grated beets in the preparation of beet kvass. When grated, beets exude too much juice resulting in a too rapid fermentation that favors the production of alcohol rather than lactic acid.

An interesting note quoted in *Nourishing Traditions:* "Professor Zabel observed that sick people always lack digestive juices, not only in the acute phase of their illness but also for a long time afterwards. In addition, he never saw a cancer victim that had a healthy intestinal flora. . . Thus, the different lacto-fermented foods are a valuable aid to the cancer patient. They are rich in vitamins and minerals and contain as well enzymes that cancer patients lack. Of particular value are lacto-fermented beets, which have a favorable effect on disturbed cellular function. Many scientific studies have demonstrated that beets have a regenerating effect on the body" (Annelies Schoneck *Des Crudités Toute L'Anneé*).

GINGER ALE
Makes 2 quarts

>*3/4 cup ginger, peeled and finely chopped or grated*
>*1/2 cup fresh lime juice*
>*1/4-1/2 cup Rapadura (see Sources)*

*2 teaspoons Celtic sea salt (see Sources)*
*1/4 cup homemade whey (pages 107-108) or 1/4 cup coconut kefir*
*2 quarts filtered water*

This is a most refreshing drink, taken in small quantities with meals and as a pick-me-up during rehearsals or practice.

Place all ingredients in a 2-quart container. Stir well and cover tightly. Leave at room temperature for 2-3 days before transferring to the refrigerator. This will keep several months well chilled.

To serve, strain into a glass. Ginger ale may be mixed with carbonated water and is best sipped at room temperature rather than gulped down cold.

Note: If you would like a naturally sparkling ginger ale, strain the ginger ale into glass bottles with wire-held stoppers or air-tight caps before transferring to the refrigerator.)

## FERMENTED VEGETABLES

Before probiotic supplements, people got their friendly bacteria by consuming lacto-fermented foods, also rich in enzymes and lactic acid, usually as condiments with cooked food.

SAUERKRAUT
Makes 1 quart

*1 medium organic cabbage, cored and shredded*
*1 tablespoon caraway seeds (optional)*
*1 tablespoon Celtic sea salt (see Sources)*
*4 tablespoons homemade whey (pages 107-108)*
*   or 1/4 cup coconut kefir (if not available,*
*   use an additional tablespoon of salt)*

In a bowl, mix the cabbage with caraway seeds, sea salt and whey. Pound mixture with a wooden pounder or meat hammer for about 10 minutes to release the juices. Place in a quart-sized, wide-mouth ma-

# 9. Recipes

son jar and press down firmly with a pounder or meat hammer until the juices come to the top of the cabbage. The top of the cabbage should be at least 1 inch below the top of the jar. Cover tightly and keep at room temperature for about three days before transferring to cold storage. The sauerkraut may be eaten immediately, but it improves with age.

PICKLED CUCUMBERS
Makes 1 quart

*4-5 pickling cucumbers*
*1 tablespoon mustard seeds*
*2 tablespoons fresh dill, snipped*
*5-6 cloves garlic (optional)*
*1 tablespoon Celtic sea salt (see Sources)*
*4 tablespoons homemade whey (pages 107-108) or coconut kefir*
    *(if not available, use an additional tablespoon of salt)*
*1 cup filtered water*

Wash cucumbers well and place them in a quart-sized, wide-mouth mason jar. Combine remaining ingredients and pour over cucumbers, adding more water if necessary to cover the cucumbers. The top of the liquid should be at least 1 inch below the top of the jar. Cover tightly and keep at room temperature for about 3 days before transferring to cold storage.

Variation: Pickled Cucumber Slices
Wash cucumbers well and slice at 1/4-inch intervals. Proceed with recipe. Pickles will be ready for cold storage after about 2 days at room temperature.

PICKLED BEETS
Makes 1 quart

> *12 medium beets*
> *seeds from 2 cardamom pods (optional)*
> *1 tablespoon Celtic sea salt*
> *4 tablespoons whey (pages 107-108) or coconut kefir*
> *(if not available, use an additional tablespoon salt)*
> *1 cup filtered water*

Prick beets in several places, place on a cookie sheet and bake at 300 degrees for about 3 hours, or until soft. Peel and cut into a ¼ - inch julienne. (Do not grate or cut the beets with a food processor— this releases too much juice, and the fermentation process will proceed too quickly, so that it favors formation of alcohol rather than lactic acid.) Place beets in a quart-sized, wide-mouth mason jar and press down lightly with a wooden pounder or hammer. Combine remaining ingredients and pour over beets, adding more water if necessary to cover the beets. The top of the beets should be at least 1 inch below the top of the jar. Cover tightly and keep at room temperature for about 3 days before transferring to cold storage.

## STOCKS

Rich stocks made from the bones of chicken, fish or beef form the basis of many delicious cuisines from around the world; stocks are also one of our most healing foods.

CHICKEN STOCK

> *1 whole pasture-raised chicken or 2-3 pounds of bony chicken parts,*
> *such as necks, backs, breastbones and wings*
> *gizzards from one chicken (optional)*
> *feet and head from the chicken (optional)*
> *4 quarts filtered water*

# 9. Recipes

*2 tablespoons apple cider vinegar*
*1 large onion, coarsely chopped*
*2-3 carrots, peeled and sliced*
*3 celery sticks, coarsely chopped*
*1 bunch parsley, tied together*

If you are using a whole chicken, cut off the wings and remove the neck, fat glands and gizzards from the cavity. By all means, use chicken feet if you can find them—they are full of gelatin. (Jewish folklore considers the addition of chicken feet the secret to successful broth.) Even better, use a whole chicken, with the head on. These may be found in Asian markets. Farm-raised, free-range chickens give the best results. Many battery-raised chickens will not produce stock that gels.

Cut chicken parts into several pieces. (If you are using a whole chicken, remove the neck and wings and cut them into several pieces.) Place chicken or chicken pieces in a large stainless steel pot with water, vinegar and all vegetables except parsley. Let stand 30 minutes to 1 hour. Bring to boil, and remove the scum that rises to the top. Reduce heat, cover and simmer for 6 to 24 hours. The longer you cook the stock, the richer and more flavorful it will be. About 10 minutes before finishing the stock, add parsley. This will impart additional minerals to the broth.

Remove whole chicken or pieces with a slotted spoon. If you are using a whole chicken, let cool and remove chicken meat from the carcass. Reserve for other uses, such as chicken salads, enchiladas, sandwiches or curries. (The skin and smaller bones, which will be very soft, may be eaten—they were traditionally consumed by cultures worldwide—or may be given to your dog or cat.) Strain the stock into a large bowl and reserve in your refrigerator until the fat rises to the top and congeals. Skim off this fat and reserve the stock in covered containers in your refrigerator or freezer.

(Note: If using a whole chicken, I often remove the chicken meat from the bones of the breast and legs as soon as it is cooked, leaving the bones, skin and meat from the bonier parts of the bird to continue to simmer. I find that when I use this meat in the final soup recipe, it is much tastier.)

BEEF STOCK

> *About 4 pounds marrowbones and knucklebones,*
>    *preferably from pastured cows*
> *1 calf's foot, cut into pieces (optional)*
> *3 pounds meaty rib or neck bones*
> *4 or more quarts cold filtered water*
> *½ cup vinegar*
> *3 onions, peeled and coarsely chopped*
> *3 carrots, peeled and coarsely chopped*
> *3 celery sticks, coarsely chopped*
> *Several sprigs fresh thyme, tied together*
> *1 teaspoon dried peppercorns, crushed*
> *1 bunch parsley, tied together*

Good beef stock must be made with several sorts of bones: knucklebones and feet impart large quantities of gelatin to the broth; marrowbones add nutrients; and meaty rib or neck bones add color and flavor.

Place the knuckle and marrowbones and optional calf's foot in a large pot with vinegar and cover with water. Let stand for one hour. Meanwhile, place the meaty bones in a roasting pan and brown at 350 degrees in the oven. When well browned, add to pot along with vegetables. Pour the fat out of the roasting pan, add cold water to the pan, set over a high flame and bring to a boil, stirring with a wooden spoon to loosen up coagulated juices. Add this liquid to the pot. Add additional water, if necessary, to cover the bones, but liquid should come no higher than one inch below the rim of the pot, as the volume expands slightly during cooking. Bring to boil. A large amount of scum will come to the top, and it is important to remove this with a spoon. After you have skimmed, reduce heat and add the thyme and crushed peppercorns.

Simmer stock for at least 12 or as long as 72 hours. Just before finishing, add the parsley and simmer another 10 minutes.

You will now have a pot of rather repulsive-looking brown liquid containing globs of gelatinous and fatty material. It doesn't even smell particularly good. But don't despair. After straining you will have a delicious and nourishing clear broth that forms the basis for many other recipes.

Remove the bones with tongs or a slotted spoon. Strain the stock into a large bowl. Let cool in the refrigerator and remove the congealed fat that rises to the top. Transfer to small containers and into the freezer for long-term storage.

FISH STOCK

> *3 or 4 whole carcasses, including heads,*
> > *of non-oily fish such as sole, turbot, rockfish or snapper*
> *2 tablespoons butter*
> *2 onions, peeled and coarsely chopped*
> *1 carrot, peeled and coarsely chopped*
> *several sprigs fresh thyme*
> *several sprigs parsley*
> *1 bay leaf*
> *1/2 cup dry white wine or vermouth*
> *1/4 cup vinegar*
> *about 3 quarts cold filtered water*

Ideally, fish stock is made from the bones of sole or turbot. In Europe, you can buy these fish on the bone. Unfortunately, in America, sole arrives at the fish market preboned. But snapper, rockfish and other non-oily fish work equally well, and a good fish merchant will save the carcasses for you if you ask him. As he normally throws these carcasses away, he shouldn't charge you for them. Be sure to take the heads as well as the body—these are especially rich in iodine and fat-soluble vitamins. Classic cooking texts advise against using oily fish such as salmon for making broth, probably because highly unsaturated fish oils become rancid during the long cooking process.

Melt the butter in a large stainless steel pot. Add the vegetables and cook very gently, about ½ hour, until they are soft. Add wine and bring to a boil. Add the fish carcasses and cover with cold, filtered water. Add vinegar. Bring to boil and skim off scum and impurities as they rise to the top. Tie herbs together and add to the pot. Reduce heat, cover and simmer for at least 4 hours or as long as 24 hours. Remove carcasses with tongs or a slotted spoon and strain the liquid into pint-sized storage containers for refrigerator or freezer. Chill well in the refrigerator and remove any congealed fat before transferring to the freezer for long-term storage.

EASY FISH BROTH: BONITO BROTH
Makes 2 quarts

> *about 1 cup shaved dried bonito (available in Asian markets)*
> *2 quarts cold filtered water*
> *1/4 cup vinegar*

This is an easy version of fish stock from Japan. Place all ingredients in a stainless steel pot, bring to boil and skim. Cover and simmer for several hours. Allow to cool and strain. Store in refrigerator or freezer.

## SOUPS

Soups from bone broths should be a daily menu element. They will help heal your digestive system and inflammatory tendencies.

# 9. Recipes

## CHICKEN OR BEEF SOUP

*2 quarts chicken or beef stock*
*2 cups meat from 1 chicken, chopped, or*
  *beef from small roast, cut into small pieces*
*6 carrots, peeled and grated*
*4 stalks celery, finely sliced*
*3 zucchini, sliced or cubed*
*2 medium onions, chopped*
*3 cloves garlic, diced (has anti-inflammatory properties)*
*2 tablespoons grated fresh ginger*
  *(has anti-inflammatory properties)*
*4 tablespoon raw butter or coconut oil*
*Celtic sea salt to taste (see Sources)*

Bring stock to gentle boil and add vegetables and butter or coconut oil, and season to taste. Cook until tender. Add chicken or beef.

Variations: Add other vegetables of your choice.

## MEDITERRANEAN FISH SOUP
(Cioppino)
Serves 8

*1-2 onions, finely chopped*
*1/4 cup extra virgin olive oil*
*6 ounces tomato paste*
*1 cup dry white wine or vermouth*
*1 1/2 quarts fish stock*
*Several sprigs fresh thyme*
*½ teaspoon oregano*
*¼ teaspoon red chile flakes*
*Pinch saffron threads*
*3 large cloves garlic, peeled and mashed*

*Celtic sea salt (see Sources) and pepper to taste*
*4 tomatoes, peeled, seeded and chopped*
*1 pound fresh sea bass, cut into cubes*
*1 pound fresh crab meat*
*1 pound fresh scallops*
*1 pound bay shrimp*
*16 fresh clams*
*8 crab claws*

Needless to say, all the seafood you use must be very fresh. You can substitute lobster for crab and mussels for clams, etc.

In a large stainless steel pot, sauté onion gently in olive oil. Stir in tomato paste and add wine, stock, spices and garlic. Bring to a rapid boil and cook vigorously, skimming occasionally, until the stock is reduced to the consistency of thin cream. Remove thyme, and season to taste. Add the seafood and tomatoes and simmer for 8-10 minutes. Ladle into large heated bowls, making sure everyone has one crab claw and two clams.

## ORGAN MEATS

Healthy traditional cultures always chose organ meats in preference to muscle meats.

CHICKEN LIVER PATÉ
Serves 12-18

*3 tablespoons butter*
*1 pound chicken or duck livers, or a combination*
*1/2 pound mushrooms, washed, dried and coarsely chopped*
*1 bunch green onions, chopped*
*2/3 cup dry white wine or vermouth*
*1 clove garlic, mashed*
*1/2 teaspoon dry mustard*
*1/4 teaspoon dried dill*

*1/4 teaspoon dried rosemary*
*1 tablespoon lemon juice*
*1/4 stick (1/4 cup) butter (preferably raw), softened*
*Celtic sea salt (see Sources)*
*Celery sticks, endive leaves or coconut crackers*

Melt butter in a heavy skillet. Add livers, onions and mushrooms and cook, stirring occasionally, for about 10 minutes, until livers are browned. Add wine, garlic, mustard, lemon juice and herbs. Bring to a boil and cook, uncovered, until the liquid is evaporated. Allow to cool. Process in a food processor with softened butter. Season to taste. Place in a crock or mold and chill well. Serve with celery sticks, endive leaves or coconut crackers.

HEARTY PATTIES
Serves 1

*1/2 cup ground beef heart*
*1/2 cup ground beef, high fat*
*1-2 tablespoon chopped onion*
*1 tablespoon parsley*
*2 tablespoons butter*
*Celtic sea salt to taste (see Sources)*

Combine ingredients and form into a patty. Lightly sauté in a skillet, rare to medium rare.

LIVER-BACON STIR FRY
Serves 2-3

*1 pound beef or calf's liver, cut into strips*
*juice of 1-2 lemons*
*1/2 pound no-nitrate bacon, cut into pieces*
*2-3 onions, peeled and sliced*

*sea salt and pepper*
*lard or extra virgin olive oil as needed*

Marinate liver strips in lemon juice several hours in the refrigerator. In a large, cast iron skillet sauté the bacon to desired crispness and move to the side of the pan. Sauté the onions in the bacon fat until golden and move to the side of the pan. Meanwhile, dry liver strips well with paper towels and season with salt and pepper. Sauté until medium rare in the pan, adding lard or olive oil as necessary. Mix bacon, onions and liver together and serve.

## EGGS
Eggs are Nature's perfect food, providing all essential amino acids in the whites and numerous important nutrients in the yolk.

## SUPER SCRAMBLE
Serves 1

*1 egg*
*1 egg yolk*
*1 tablespoon cream*
*1 tablespoon butter*
*1 teaspoon chopped parsley (optional)*
*Celtic sea salt to taste (see Sources)*

Beat egg, egg yolk, cream, salt and parsley. Cook gently in butter.

## CHEESE OMELET
Serves 1

*2 eggs*
*1 tablespoon water*
*Celtic sea salt to taste (see Sources)*
*dash tabasco sauce*

*1/2 cup raw grated cheddar*
*1 tablespoon butter*

Beat eggs with water, salt and tabasco sauce. Melt butter in a cast iron skillet. When it foams, add the egg mixture. Sprinkle cheese on top. After a few minutes, fold the omelet in half. Remove from heat but let sit a minute before serving so the center cooks through.

## NUT SNACKS
Although nuts are touted as excellent snack foods, they are hard to digest because nature provides them with enzyme inhibitors that keep them from sprouting. Therefore, if you eat quantities of nuts, they may upset your stomach and irritate your mouth. Traditional cultures understood the principle that nuts are digested best when soaked or partially sprouted before eating. This also makes their nutrients more readily available.

## CRISPY PECANS, WALNUTS, CASHEWS OR ALMONDS
Makes 4 cups

*4 cups raw pecans, walnut halves, cashews or almonds*
   *(preferably skinless)*
*2 teaspoons Celtic sea salt (see Sources)*
*filtered water*

Mix pecans, walnuts, cashews or almonds with salt and cover with filtered water. Leave in a warm place for 7 to 8 hours or overnight. (Note: Soak cashews no more than 6 hours.) Drain in colander. Spread nuts on a stainless steel baking pan and place in a warm oven (no more than 150 degrees) for 12 to 24 hours, turning occasionally, until completely dry and crisp. (You may also use a dehydrator.) Store in an airtight container. Cashews, almonds and pecans may be stored at room temperature, but walnuts should be stored in the refrigerator.

GLUTEN-FREE NUT CRACKERS
Makes 16-20
> *2 1/2 cups raw walnuts or skinless almonds*
> *2 tablespoons Celtic sea salt (see Sources)*
> *1 small onion, coarsely chopped*
> *1 tablespoon fresh minced rosemary, thyme or garlic*
> *2 teaspoons raw red wine or apple cider vinegar*
> *1 tablespoon honey*
> *1 teaspoon Celtic sea salt (see Sources)*

Soak almonds or walnuts overnight in filtered water mixed with 2 tablespoons Celtic sea salt. Drain in a colander. Place in a food processor along with remaining ingredients. Process to form a coarse paste. Spread mixture as thin as possible onto cookie sheets lined with buttered parchment paper. Place a sheet of parchment paper over the paste and roll thin with a rolling pin. Score with a knife into cracker-sized squares. Dehydrate in a warm oven (preferably at 150 degrees) for 12-24 hours until completely dry. Adopted from *Recipes for Life* by Becky Mauldin.

## WHOLE GRAINS

Here are a few recipes that will give you experience with the proper preparation of grains. You may try these recipes after a period of abstinence from grains. If you have no reaction to eating grains after this period, you may be able to enjoy small amounts of properly prepared grains. These are wonderful examples of ways you can incorporate grains into your diet in a traditionally nutritious manner. As you will see, soaking grains in whey, kefir, yogurt or buttermilk (or, if you have allergies to milk, in coconut kefir or water mixed with a little vinegar or lemon juice), for at least 7 hours is a standard preparation technique that will break down phytic acid and enzyme inhibitors.

## 9. Recipes

BREAKFAST PORRIDGE
Serves 4

> *1 cup rolled oats*
> *1 cup warm filtered water plus 2 tablespoons whey (pages 107-108),*
> *raw milk yogurt, kefir or buttermilk, or coconut kefir, lemon juice or*
> *vinegar (if you have allergies to milk)*
> *1/2 teaspoon Celtic sea salt (see Sources)*
> *1 cup filtered water*
> *1 tablespoon flax seeds, freshly ground (optional)*

For highest benefits and best assimilation, porridge should be soaked overnight or even longer. Once soaked, oatmeal cooks up in less than 5 minutes—truly a *fast food*.

Mix oats with warm water mixture, cover and leave in a warm place for at least 7 hours or as long as 24 hours. Bring an additional cup of water to boil with sea salt. Add soaked oats, reduce heat, cover and simmer several minutes. Meanwhile, grind the flax seeds in a mini grinder. Remove from heat, stir in optional flax seeds and let stand for a few minutes. Serve with plenty of butter or cream and a natural sweetener like Rapadura, date sugar, maple syrup, maple sugar or raw honey.

BROWN RICE
Serves 6-8

> *2 cups long-grain or short-grain rice*
> *4 cups warm filtered water plus 4 tablespoons whey (pages 107-108),*
> *raw milk yogurt, kefir or buttermilk, or coconut kefir, lemon juice or*
> *vinegar (if you have allergies to milk)*
> *1 teaspoon Celtic sea salt (see Sources)*
> *2-4 tablespoons butter*

Place rice and warm water mixture in a flameproof casserole and leave in a warm place for at least 7 hours. Bring to boil, skim, reduce heat, stir in salt and butter and cover tightly. Without removing lid, cook over lowest possible heat for about 45 minutes.

COCONUT CRACKERS
About 40 crackers

If you have time to make your own crackers, these will be superior to anything you can buy in the store. Unfortunately, as of this writing, there is no brand of commercial crackers made with coconut oil. Please note that this recipe may be problematical for those with gluten allergies.

> *2 1/2 cups freshly ground spelt, kamut, whole-wheat, or rye,*
> *    or a mixture*
> *1 cup plain yogurt*
> *1 teaspoon Celtic sea salt (see Sources)*
> *1 1/2 teaspoons baking powder*
> *1/2 cup melted coconut oil*
> *arrowroot powder*

Mix flour with yogurt and leave in a warm place for 24 hours. Preheat oven to 200 degrees Place soaked flour, salt, baking powder, and 1/4 cup coconut oil in a food processor and process until well blended. Roll out to about 1/16 inch on a pastry cloth dusted with arrowroot to prevent sticking. Cut into 2-inch squares with a knife. Place on an oiled cookie sheet, brush with remaining 1/4 cup coconut oil, and bake in oven (or dehydrator) for several hours, or until completely dry and crisp. Store in an airtight container.

## 10

# THE BODY IN BALANCE

*A*n optimally nourished body is resilient. However, in maintaining this resiliency, your spiritual health and physical fitness play vital roles. If any one of these foundations of health is out of balance or ignored, the whole body will be affected.

Taking care of your spirit helps you balance the daily stresses you encounter in relationships, busy schedules and demanding careers, while fulfilling your high performance standards. It is extremely beneficial to spend some time each day in a quiet place where you can "recharge your batteries." Something as simple as 10-30 minutes daily doing meditation, using deep abdominal breathing and focusing on positive thoughts, can invigorate each day with a fresh outlook. Practicing deep breathing, self soothing and positive affirmations throughout the day will strengthen your ability to focus on the best of each moment. Becoming "stressed-out" does not happen overnight! Even the healthiest diet won't protect you against the effects of stress if you ignore the need to be centered and strong in your spirit.

Consider the fact that the digestion process is directly connected to emotional responses. For instance, when you are upset or agitated, your digestion may become upset as well—you may even experience loose bowels or diarrhea. Under these circumstances, the foods that you are digesting are moving at a quicker pace through your digestive tract, and their nutrients may not be absorbed as thoroughly as they should. You may also find that the use of your muscles for your work becomes very difficult. Thus, for optimal digestion, assimilation and muscle strength, balancing emotional responses to stress with meditation and deep breathing will help your body better utilize the nutrients from your foods and enhance fine muscle control.

Dr. Turner discusses the important fact that optimal health is not the absence of disease, but a balance of the physical, biochemical and emotional aspects of our being. If any one aspect is stressed, the others will be affected.

An example of this principle is the blushing of the face when you are angry or embarrassed. The dilation of the blood vessels in the face is a physical and physiologic reaction to a purely emotional trigger.

Similar reactions occur in the gut in response to emotions. Have you ever heard of a "gut feeling"? Even without knowing about the physiology of the body's reaction to emotional stress, mankind has an inherent awareness of this interwoven connection.

Canadian researcher Hans Selye demonstrated through solid research the specific reactions of the body to stress, whether it be physical, biochemical or emotional in origin. One of these reactions is an impairment of the digestive process. Poor digestion results in poor nutrient absorption and ultimately diminished energy, both mentally and physiologically—inconsequential if the stress is short-lived but extremely debilitating when endured over the longterm.

Another reaction caused by stress is the inhibition of secretory IgA (SIgA) production by the mucous lining of the intestines. SIgA is our first line of defense against a host of invading viruses and organisms trying to enter our bodies through the GI tract. Imagine how long it would take some opportunistic invader to enter your home if you went on vacation and left all your windows and doors wide open!

Lastly, reactions to stress can cause a reduction in peripheral circulation, resulting in decreased blood flow to the arms and legs. Musicians, dancers and athletes require optimal levels of blood flow for prolonged muscle energy. Balancing stress will therefore help you perform at your best.

A strong physical fitness level is essential to optimal health; physical activity is also another excellent way to balance stress. Athletes and dancers are always in motion on the job, but musicians, keyboard operators and those whose work is sedentary often spend long hours in the same position each day. Consistently taking the time for both cardiovascular and muscle-balancing exercise is critical to maintaining a feeling of well-being. For those who sit for long hours, exercises that strengthen the lower back and core muscles can be very effective in reducing stress—as can a daily walk in the out of doors.

Maintaining true health is an ongoing process of integration, of maintaining nutritional, physical and spiritual balance. You can benefit by fine-tuning your individual needs in all of these areas.

# SOURCES

Alcohol-Free (Gluten-Free) Extracts: Frontier (800) 669-3275; frontierherb.com; and in health food stores.

Breads: Sourdough breads made with Celtic sea salt can be ordered from Mountain Eagle Bakery (406) 222-3617; Grain & Salt Society (800) 867-7258; or Miller's Bakery (530) 532-6384.

Butter, Grass-Fed and High-Vitamin: See classified ads in *Wise Traditions,* journal of the Weston A. Price Foundation (202) 363-4394, westonaprice.org.

Butter Oil, High-Vitamin (X-Factor): Radiant Life (888) 593-8333, radiantlifecatalog.com; Dr. Ron's Ultra-Pure (877) 472-8701, drrons.com; Green Pastures (402) 338-5551, greenpasture.org.

Celtic Sea Salt: Grain & Salt Society (800) 867-7258; Radiant Life (888) 593-8333, radiantlifecatalog.com.

Clarified Butter (Ghee): Purity Farms Ghee (from pastured cows), available in health food stores.

Coconut, Creamed: Tropical Traditions, 866-311-2626, tropicaltraditions.com; Asian and Indian food shops.

Coconut Milk, whole and full fat (organic): in health food stores; for a superior coconut milk concentrate, called "natural coconut cream," coconutoil-online.com, (800) 922-1744.

Coconut Oil: Tropical Traditions (866) 311-2626, tropicaltraditions.com; Radiant Life (888) 593-8333, radiantlifecatalog.com; coconutoil-online.com (800) 922-1744; Wilderness Family Naturals (866) 936-6457, wildernessfamilynaturals.com; Green Pastures (402) 338-5551, greenpasture.org.

Cod Liver Oil: High-vitamin cod liver oil from Radiant Life (888) 593-8333, radiantlifecatalog.com; Dr. Ron's Ultra-Pure (877) 472-8701; drrons.com; Green Pastures (402) 338-5551, greenpasture.org. Regular strength cod liver oil from Garden of Life, in health food stores.

Colostrum: Immune Tree colostrum available from Radiant Life (888) 593-8333, radiantlifecatalog.com.

Dolomite Powder (Calcium Carbonate): KAL brand (800) 634-1380, needs.com.

Enzymes: Radiant Life (888) 593-8333, radiantlifecatalog.com.

Fermented Raw Vegetables: Rejuvenative Foods (800) 805-7957; www.rejuvenative.com; Goldmine sauerkraut (858) 537-9830; Real Pickles (413) 863-9063.

Ghee (Clarified Butter): Purity Farms Ghee (from pastured cows), available in health food stores.

## Sources

Grain Mills: Jupiter grain mill may be ordered from New Market Naturals (800) 873-4321, newmarketnaturals.com; other mills are available from Lehman's (877) 438-5346; or with other attachments (slicer, meat grinder) from Radiant Life (888) 593-8333, radiantlifecatalog.com.

Honey, Raw: Really Raw Honey (800) REALRAW; Garden of Life, in health food stores

Kefir Powder: Body Ecology (866) 533-4748, bodyecologydiet.com.

Kombucha: Ready-made kombucha and kits for making kombucha available through kombucha2000.com, (877) 566-2824. GT'S Organic Raw Kombucha available in health food stores or through GTSkombucha.com, (877) 735-8423.

Maple Syrup (organic, non-formaldehyde): Grain & Salt Society (800) 867-7258; Coombs Vermont Gourmet (888) 266-6271, maplesource.com.

Meat-Pasture-Raised: See classified ads in *Wise Traditions,* journal of the Weston A. Price Foundation (202) 363-4394, or contact a local chapter, listed at WestonAPrice/org/localchapters; see also eatwild.com.

Milk, Raw: Visit realmilk.com or contact a local chapter of the Weston A. Price Foundation, listed at WestonAPrice.org/localchapters, (202) 333-HEAL.

Miso: South River Miso Company (413) 369-4057, southrivermiso.com; Gold Mine Natural Foods (858) 537-9830, goldminenaturalfood.com

Olive Oil (unrefined, organic, extra virgin): Pietro del Marco (914) 723-5850; Bariani Olive Oil from Radiant Life (888) 593-8333, radiantlifecatalog.com.

Perfect Food Supplement: Garden of Life, in health food stores, or call Living Springs (800) 520-1791, thelivingspring.com.

Rapadura: (800) 207-2814, rapunzel.com; or in health food stores.

Super Greens SBO Supplement: Super Greens and Dunaliella available through Radiant Life (888) 593-8333, radiantlifecatalog.com.

Sourdough Bread Cultures: G.E.M. Cultures (707) 964-2922, www.gemcultures.com.

Soy Sauce, naturally fermented: South River Miso Company (413) 369-4057; Ohsawa Nama Shoyu unpasteurized soy sauce, in health food stores.

Spices, Herbs (nonirradiated), Alcohol-Free Extracts: Frontier (800) 669-3275, frontierherb.com; and in health food stores.

Vitamin Supplements, additive-free: Dr. Ron's Ultra-Pure (877) 472-8701, drrons.com.

Yogurt:  Good brands of whole plain yogurt available commercially include Traderspoint, Seven Stars Farm, Brown Cow and Butterworks.

## *Sources*

### THE WESTON A. PRICE FOUNDATION

The Weston A. Price Foundation was founded in 1999 to disseminate the research of nutrition pioneer Weston A. Price, DDS, whose studies of isolated nonindustrialized peoples established the parameters of human health and determined the optimum characteristics of human diets. Dr. Price's research demonstrated that humans achieve perfect physical form and perfect health generation after generation only when they consume nutrient-dense whole foods and the vital fat-soluble activators found exclusively in animal fats.

The Foundation is dedicated to restoring nutrient-dense foods to the American diet through education, research and activism and supports a number of movements that contribute to this objective, including accurate nutrition instruction, organic and biodynamic farming, pasture feeding of livestock, community supported farms, honest and informative labeling, prepared parenting and nurturing therapies.

Local chapters of the Foundation help people find organic and farm-raised foods in their locality, particularly meats, eggs and dairy foods from animals on pasture.

The Foundation's quarterly journal, *Wise Traditions in Food, Farming and the Healing Arts,* is dedicated to exploring the scientific validation of dietary, agricultural and healing traditions throughout the world. It features illuminating and thought-provoking articles on current scientific research; human diets; nontoxic agriculture; and holistic therapies. The journal also serves as a source for foods that have been conscientiously grown and processed.

For subscription, chapter and membership information contact:

The Weston A. Price Foundation
PMB 106-380, 4200 Wisconsin Avenue, NW
Washington, DC 20016
(202) 363-4394
website: www.WestonAPrice.org   email: info@westonaprice.org

# *Website and Seminar Information*

Dr. John Turner and Kathryne Pirtle are available for seminars on building optimal health through traditional food. They have presented engaging Power Point presentations to orchestras, dance companies, university music and dance schools, athletic teams and the general public. These presentations advance an understanding of the necessary nutritional elements that help heal chronic ailments and promote a higher level of health, which ensure career longevity and a higher quality of life.

Topics include:

Optimal Nutrition for Performance and Career Longevity
(for performers)

Recovering from Malnutrition Associated with
Digestive Disorders (for the general public)

Building Optimal Health with Traditional Foods
(for the general public)

For seminar information: Visit
www.performancewithoutpain.com

To schedule a seminar: Contact Kathryne Pirtle at
kathypirtle@sbcglobal.net

# INDEX

# Index

# Related Titles from NewTrends Publishing

NOURISHING TRADITIONS
*The Cookbook that Challenges
Politically Correct Nutrition and the Diet Dictocrats*
by Sally Fallon and Mary G. Enig, PhD

THE CHOLESTEROL MYTHS
*Exposing the Fallacy that Saturated Fat
and Cholesterol Cause Heart Disease*
by Uffe Ravnskov, MD, PhD

THE YOGA OF EATING
*Transcending Diets and Dogma
to Nourish the Natural Self*
by Charles Eisenstein

THE UNTOLD STORY OF MILK
*Green Pastures, Contented Cows and Raw Dairy Foods*
by Ron Schmid, ND

THE FOURFOLD PATH TO HEALING
*Working with the Laws of Nutrition, Therapeutics,
Movement and Meditation in the Art of Medicine*
by Thomas S. Cowan, MD
with Sally Fallon and Jaimen McMillan

THE WHOLE SOY STORY
*The Dark Side of America's Favorite Health Food*
by Kaayla T. Daniel, PhD

HONORING OUR CYCLES
*A Natural Family Planning Workbook
For Knowing which Days You Can and Can't Get Pregnant*
by Katie Singer

To order, call (877) 707-1776
or visit www.newtrendspublishing.com.

# ABOUT THE AUTHORS

KATHRYNE PIRTLE is the clarinetist and executive director of the critically acclaimed Orion Ensemble, which tours throughout North America, presents three series each year in the Chicago metropolitan area, and performs a live, internationally broadcast series on WFMT, Fine Arts Radio in Chicago. She is Principal Clarinetist of the Lake Forest Symphony, and frequently performs with the Lyric Opera, Grant Park Symphony, Ravinia Festival Orchestra and the Chicago Symphony. In addition, she has served on the faculties of the Wheaton College Conservatory and Northern Illinois University. In 2004, the Hal Leonard Corporation released her solo album of selected Bach unaccompanied cello and violin suites and sonatas transcribed for the clarinet by Himie Voxman.

SALLY FALLON is the author of the best-selling *Nourishing Traditions: The Cookbook that Challenges Politically Correct Nutrition and the Diet Dictocrats*. This thought-provoking guide to traditional foods contains a startling message: Animal fats and cholesterol are not villains but vital factors in the diet, necessary for normal growth, proper function of the brain and nervous system and protection from disease. She is a founding president of the Weston A. Price Foundation and editor of the Foundation's quarterly magazine, as well as the founder of A Campaign for Real Milk. *Eat Fat Lose Fat* (Penguin, Hudson Street Press), by Sally Fallon and Dr. Mary Enig, was published in December 2004.

JOHN D. TURNER, DC, CCSP, DIBCN was a national qualifying gymnast, an experience that inspired his life-long passion in the field of health. A trained chiropractor, he has postgraduate certification in acupuncture and sports medicine. Because of his unique qualifications, he has been commissioned to serve on the medical staff at a number of Big Ten Track and Field Championships, the U.S. Track and Field Championships and the U.S. and World Gymnastics Championships.